FEMALE GENITAL ANATOMIC DEVIATIONS: FROM EMBRYOGENESIS TO SURGERY

Female genital anatomic deviations: from embryogenesis to surgery

By Dr. Zohrab Makiyan

Copyright © 2023 Zograb Makiyan
First Edition
Standard Copyright License
All rights reserved
ISBN – 978-1-387-15970-3
Published on January 2023
Language English
Autor Spotlight URL:
http://www.lulu.com/spotlight/Zohrab

This work is licensed under the
Creative Commons Attribution-ShareAlike 3.0 Unported License To view a copy of this license, visit:
http://creativecommons.org/license/by-nc/2.5/
or send a letter to:
Creative Commoms
171mSecond Street, Suite 300
San Francisco, California 94105»

CONTENTS

FEMALE GENITAL ANATOMIC DEVIATIONS: FROM EMBRYOGENESIS TO SURGERY 1
CONTENTS 3
PREFACE 5
BACKGROUND 7
I. GONADAL SEX DIFFERENTIATION 11
    Testis 11
    Ovary 12
    Surgery 13
    Conclusions 24
    A new hypothesis to describe gonadal embryogenesis 25
    References 32
II. UTEROVAGINAL ANATOMIC DEVIATIONS 35
    Introduction 35
    Results 37
    Discussion 56
    References 60
III. NEW THEORY OF UTEROVAGINAL EMBRYOGENESIS ... 63
    Introduction 63
    Clinical evidences 65
    Experimental evidences 67
    Discussion 73
    References 77

IV. ENDOMETRIUM ORIGINATING FROM PRIMORDIAL GERM CELLS 81
    Introduction 81
    Endometriosis theories 83
    Germ cells in embryo 86
    New theory of endometriosis origination from primordial germ cells 87
    Speculations about the etiology of endometriosis with clinical evidence supporting the new theory 90
    Conclusion 95
    References 97

V. AMBIGUOUS EXTERNAL GENITALIA 101
    Introduction 101
    Materials and methods 104
    Results 104
    Discussion 121
    Speculation about the derivation of the genital tubercle 126
    References 132

VI. SYSTEMATIZATION FOR FEMALE GENITAL VARIATIONS 135

VII. NEW INSIGHTS INTO THE EMBRYOGENESIS OF THE FEMALE REPRODUCTIVE SYSTEM 139
    Clinical and experimental evidences 144
    Conclusion 147
    References 149
    Abbreviations 151

Front cover art image 152
Author page 153

Epygraph: *Anomaly or Diversity of Nature?*

PREFACE

Congenital anatomic (structural) deviations (variations) of the reproductive system arise during embryonal organogenesis, although their clinical manifestations present later in newborns or in adolescence and during reproductive years due to functional disorders, abnormal menstruation, sexual dysfunction, infertility and pregnancy loss.

The aim of this paper is to distinguish female genital anatomic variations for appropriate surgical treatment based on a clinical analysis. Surgical treatment of congenital variations is performed according to variant anatomy and functional disorders. However, many congenital anatomic variations are difficult to categorize based on current classification systems.

Medical records were reviewed for surgical treatments of 1320 cases of uterovaginal malformation and 235 cases with disorders of sex development. between 1998 and 2022 at the National Medical Research Center for Obstetrics, Gynecology, and Perinatology in Moscow, Russia.

Physical variations were assessed by ultrasound, magnetic resonance imaging, and laparoscopy. Genetic studies were conducted for individuals with disorders of sex development. Classification of anatomic variants was determined by physical findings, genetic findings, and clinical presentations.

A unified Systematization for Female Genital Anatomic Variations was proposed, based on the genome (karyotype), gonadal morphology, internal and external genital anatomy. The internal anatomy was classified to uterovaginal variations, which have distinguished to 11 basic types and 24 variants, according to morphologic patterns. Surgical treatments are proposed based on these variants.

These new classifications provide a framework for clinical management and appropriate surgical treatment of female uterovaginal anatomic variants, with the aim of improving reproductive outcomes.

Genital structural anomalies are defined as deviations from normal anatomy resulting of embryological maldevelopment. The clinical anatomy of the structural variations, were observed according to the embryonic developmental stages. A systematic comparison of reproductive organ anatomic variations (malformations) with contemporary embryological investigations and literature reviews revealed that many controversies exist, stimulating the formulation of a new concept of embryonic morphogenesis. Here, this new systematic view of the reproductive system morphogenesis, the controversies surrounding it, and evidence-based arguments in its favour are being discussed.

The new theories have been proposed the significant conceptual changes about: uterovaginal development from mesonephral ducts; gonadal morphogenesis and development of genital tubercle from sacral somytes.

I believe, the proposed theories may be useful for future embryological investigations, especially for understanding the dual origin of the uterine folds from fused mesonephric ducts with gonadal ridges.

Lots of researches devoted to the study of ectopic endometriosis, but derivation of eutopic (normally cited) endometrium is still unknown.

It may be the key for understanding the aetiology of female genital anomalies and major benign gynaecological diseases, comma leiomyoma and enigmantic endometriosis from polypotential germ cells.

BACKGROUND

According to current views, reproductive systems develop through consecutive developmental stages: genetic, gonadal and hormonal, followed by internal and external organ morphogenesis (Cunha et al 2017; Fritsch et al 2013; Hill 2019a; Jost 1972; Muller 1830; Nistal et al 2007; Sadler 2004; Tschopp et al. 2014; Wilhelm et al. 2007).

Initially, the genital system consists of gonads or primitive sex glands, genital ducts, and indifferent external genitalia that will differentiate either through the male or female pathways (Batista 2019; Hill 2019a; Jost 1972; Nistal et al 2007; Sadler 2004; Robboy et al 2017; Tschopp et al. 2014; Wilhelm et al. 2007):

1. At the genetic stage, chromosomal sex is established at fertilization: chromosomes XY indicate males; and XX denote females.

2. The germline epithelium of indifferent gonads originates from primordial germ cells that migrate by an amoeboid movement from the yolk sac through the peritoneum to the dorsolateral gonadal ridges at an early developmental stage.

3. Gonadal differentiation depends on SRY gene persistence. During this period, indifferent gonads develop either into testes (SRY-positive genome) or ovaries (SRY-negative genome).

   The mechanism by which *SRY*-negative specification leads to ovary development is unknown. This is unclear: why do SRY-negative ovotesticular patients with a 46,XX karyotype have testicular components in their gonads; and why do the SRY-negative patients (in 46,XX-male syndrome) have testes?

   The embryonal pathogenesis of ambiguous gonads (ovotestis) inexplicable.

4. At the hormonal stage, sex differentiation depends upon the testosterone-influenced virilization of the mesonephric ducts, urogenital sinus, and external genitalia.

   By the 8th week of gestation in male embryos, the Leydig cells of the testes begin to produce testosterone and induce sexual differentiation of both the genital ducts and external genitalia into male characteristics. Simultaneously, the Müllerian-Inhibiting Substance (MIS) or the anti-Müllerian hormone (AMH) induce the regression of the Müllerian ducts.

   According to Jost's (Jost 1972) theory, in the absence or inactivity of testicular hormones, the indifferent organs develop following the female pathway.

   Due to gonadal differentiation the internal genitalia develop into male or female pathway.

   How do some 46,XY DSD patients develop Mullerian ducts derivatives, including Fallopian tubes, uterine rudiments? It is currently unknown.

5. Müller (1830) described two pairs of internal genital ducts: one, located medially just below the gonadal ridges (growing caudally), corresponding to the mesonephric ducts (Wolffian). The other one, corresponding to the paramesonephric ducts (Müllerian), develops autonomously to the paramedial zone of the mesonephric ducts.

   In the male pathway, the mesonephric derivatives persist and form the main excretory genital ducts - the seminiferous tubules, the efferent ductules, which conjoin to the rete testis and develop into the testicular ductuli deferentes (respectively). Whereas the sustentacular cells of Sertoli are derived from the mesonephric excretory tubules, the interstitial Leydig cells are derived from the original mesenchyme of the mesonephros. The mesonephric tubules have an inductive influence over the primordial gonads (germ cells) to drive their development into testes.

In the female pathway, the paramesonephric ducts form the fallopian tubes, the uterus, and the vagina. The uterus develops by the fusion of the Müllerian ducts together and the reduction of the intermedial septum in a craniocaudal direction. The mesonephric ducts completely regress in the female embryo.

According to Mullerian theory, the mesonephric ducts do not intersect with paramesonephric ducts anywhere, because they growing at the different parallel parts. How explain, that female reproductive tract, which is growing by symmetric fusion of two identical Mullerian ducts, then differentiates into uterine folds with large myometrial layer and endometrial cavity. A lot of scientists investigate the ectopic endometrium, but where is it from derivation of the normally cited endometrium? That is a grate question.

6. The external genitalia in both sexes develop from the genital tubercle, the genital swellings, and the genital folds (from the 3rd to the 12th week of embryonic development).

The genital tubercle is the embryonic progenitor of penis and clitoris. According to current views, the genital tubercle originates from mesenchymal tissue, but mesenchymal cells are arranged across the embryonic body and do not have specific androgen receptors (Tschopp et al. 2014; Herrera and Cohn 2014).

The genital swellings rise on each side of the urethral folds to form the scrotal buds in males and the labia majora in females. The nature of the signals that initiate the early derivation of the indifferent genital tubercle is currently unknown (Tschopp et al. 2014).

Why do androgens cause virilization influence on the indifferent genital tubercle, and why does this hormonal influence promote the outgrowth and elongation of the clitoris (on female embryo) or penis (on male embryo)?

I. GONADAL SEX DIFFERENTIATION

At the genetic stage, chromosomal sex is established at fertilization in which XY indicates male and XX denotes female. During the first two months of human gestation, the two sexes develop identically. The gonadal stage is the period during which indifferent gonads develop into either ovaries or testes. The phenotypic stage is induced in response to gonadal differentiation; the internal genital tract and external genitalia develop into characteristic male or female structures. [1-4]

Gonads appear initially as a pair of longitudinal genital or gonadal ridges at the 4-5th week. Primitive gonads are formed by the proliferation of germ cells, which migrate from the yolk sac and undergo condensation of the underlying mesenchyme in the sixth week. The gonads do not acquire male or female morphological characteristics until the seventh week of development, so they are classified as indifferent. [1-4]

Mesonephros is primary embryonal kidney, which functions for a short time during the early fetal period (in the fourth week). The mesonephros and mesonephric ducts are derived from intermediate mesoderm. In the 6th week, the mesonephros forms a large ovoid organ on each side of the midline, which is lateral to the gonadal ridges. Laterally, the tubule enters the longitudinal collecting ducts, which are known as the mesonephric ducts. In male embryos, some caudal tubules and the mesonephric ducts persist and participate in the formation of the genital system, while they disappear in females. [1-3]

Testis

If an embryo is genetically male (46,XY), the indifferent gonad differentiates to testes under influence of the SRY gene on the Y chromosome, which encodes testis-determining factor. The primitive proliferating sex cords penetrate deep into the gonadal medulla to form the medullary cords of the testis. Testis cords are composed of primitive germ cells and sustentacular cells of Sertoli derived from the surface epithelium of the mesonephral ducts.

Interstitial Leydig cells, which are derived from the original mesenchyme of the gonadal ridge, lie between the testis cords.

The mesonephric ducts persist and form the main genital ducts of male embryo. The efferent ductules represent the remaining parts of the mesonephric system excretory tubules. These link the rete testis and mesonephric duct, which become the ductus deferens. The seminiferous tubules join to the rete testis tubules, which in turn enter into the ductuli efferentes. [1-4]

Ovary

In female embryos with a 46,XX sex chromosome complement, primitive sex cords dissociate into irregular cell clusters. These clusters, which contain groups of primitive germ cells, occupy the medullary part of the ovary. Later, they disappear and are replaced by a vascular stroma that forms the ovarian medulla. These cords split into isolated cell clusters, which each surround one or more primitive germ cells. Germ cells subsequently develop into oogonia, while the surrounding epithelial cells, descendants of the surface epithelium, form follicular cells. [1-4]

According to Alfred Jost (1976), sex differentiation depends upon testosterone influenced virilization on the mesonephral ducts, urogenital sinus and external genitalia. Jost resolved the controversy surrounding the mechanism of somatic sex differentiation by establishing that male characteristics must be imposed on the fetus by the testicular hormones testosterone and MIS, respectively, which are responsible for the virilization of the mesonephral ducts, urogenital sinus and external genitalia as well as for regression of the Mullerian ducts. [4] In the absence or inactivity of these hormones, the development of the fetus is stalled at an indifferent stage; thus, it becomes phenotypically female. By the eighth week of gestation, Leydig cells of the testes begin to produce testosterone and the testes can influence sexual differentiation of the genital ducts and external genitalia. Formation of the external genitalia is completed by the 12th week. [1-4]

Surgery

Disorders of sex development (DSD) are congenital conditions in which chromosomal, gonadal, or anatomical sex development is atypical. [5-15]
Epidemiological studies have estimated a rate of 2.2 per 10,000 cases with ambiguous genitalia in newborns. [16]

All DSD patients were classified into three categories that were based on karyotype: with sex chromosome anomalies, with male karyotype 46,XY DSD, and female karyotype 46,XX DSD. For a review see refs. [7-14]

Management and surgical correction were performed according to the Guidelines of European Consensus Statement in DSD, 2006, 2010, and 2018. For a review see refs. [5-11]

Clinical assessments included karyotyping, ultrasound imaging, hormone measurements and investigations of gonadal morphology. All individuals received a female gender assignment after clinical investigations.

Surgical correction for female patients with DSD included laparoscopic gonadal biopsy (46,XX; 45,X/46,XX) or adnexectomy in XY karyotype patients. [13]

Feminizing clitoroplasty was performed for patients with ambiguous genitalia (in severe III–IV degrees of virilization by Prader). [14]

Females with AIS and classic Turner syndrome underwent creation of a neovagina.

Gonad removal was performed in female patients with androgen insensitivity syndrome (AIS); 46,XY gonadal dysgenesis, SRY-positive and ovotesticular DSD, to prevent the development of malignancy in adulthood.

Gonadal biopsy allowed for verification of ovarian dysgenesis or streak-gonads in SRY-negative patients with X-monosomy and chimerism. For a review see refs. [6-13]

Investigations of gonadal morphology revealed patterns that were related to established types of gonadal dysgenesis.

Turner syndrome is caused by partial or complete loss of one of the two X chromosomes or mosaics of 45,X cells with 46,XX cells, 46,XY, or other karyotypes (e.g., cells bearing 46,XdelXp, 46,XiXq). In Turner females, the frequency of mosaicism is estimated to range from 67% to 90%. [17]

The three fibrous streak types of the gonads distinguished in patients with Turner syndrome [13]:

> Classical fibrous streak-gonads, with a 45,X karyotype. The whitish streak gonads, which histologically contain fibrous tissue, contain no ovarian follicles.
>
> Utero-vaginal aplasia can be detected during laparoscopy. The Mullerian ducts derivates – Fallopian tubes.

> The fibrous streak-gonads with occasional ovarian follicles, presenting as ovarian dysgenesis revealed by a 45,X/46,XX mosaic karyotype. The ovaries appear hypoplastic with a higher degree of X-monosomy. In other cases with a prevalence of normal 46,XX cells, they present with an anatomically and functionally normal ovary.
>
> They also present with a hypoplastic normal shaped uterus and vagina.

> The fibrous streak cord at one gonadal pole and testicular tissue in another, can occur in a patient with 45,X/46,XY mosaicism. The streak pole contains only fibrous tissue without oocytes; the testicular pole contains a dysgenetic structure

with anastomosed tubular formations, such as streak-testes (Fig. I-1a, b).

In cases in which oocytes are present, the patient is defined as ovotesticular DSD.

These patients had persistent Mullerian ducts derivates (PMDS – persistent Mullerian syndrome): Fallopian tubes and uterine rudiments.

Figure I-1a. Patient with 45,X/46,XY mosaicism, laparoscopy.

The right gonad contains a whitish fibrous streak cord and dysgenetic testicular structure. Persistent Mullerian ducts derivates detected: Fallopian tube, rudimental uterus.

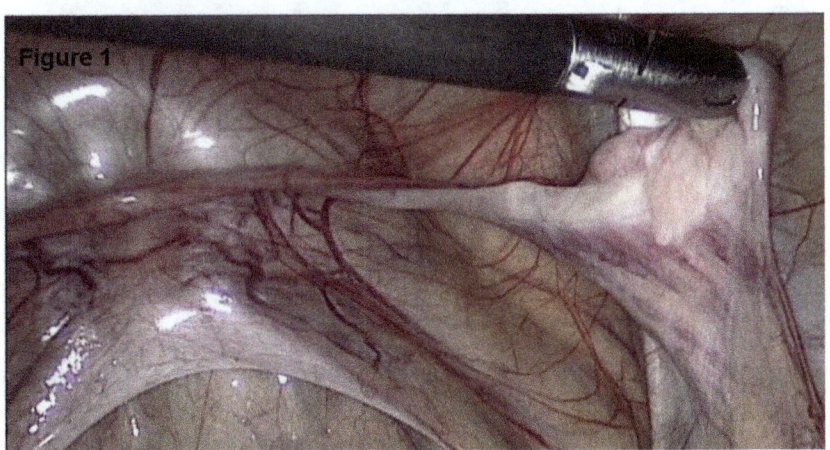

Figure I-1b. Fibrous-streak gonad.

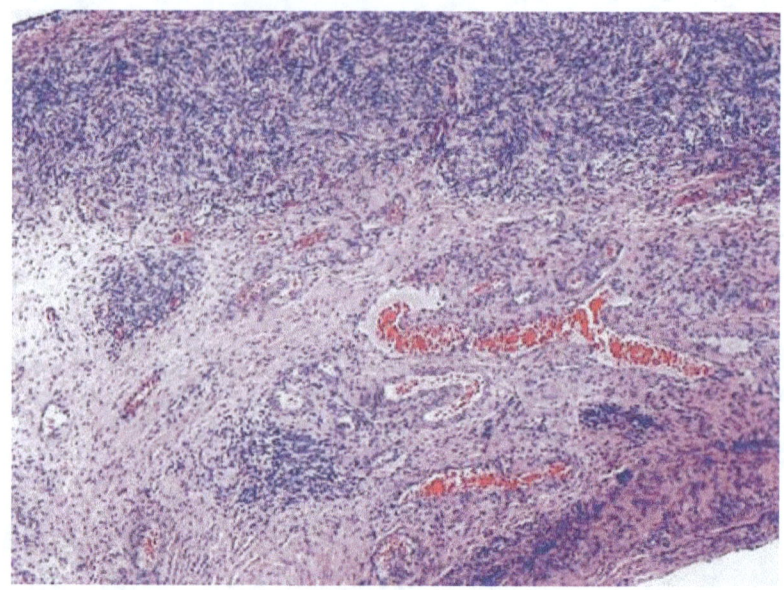

Normally, the SRY gene encodes the sex-determining region Y-protein, which is a transcription factor of the testis-determining protein family that initiates male sex determination. Mutation of SRY prevents testes differentiation, resulting gonadal dysgenesis. [4, 12, 15]

Patients with 46,XY testicle dysgenesis are characterized by a reduced tubular diameter and an increased presence of Sertoli cells in both gonads.

- Patients with the complete form without virilization of the external genitalia (i.e., completely feminine) had a normal shaped hypoplastic uterus, Fallopian tubes and vagina.

- In the incomplete form, patients are characterized by ambiguous genitalia resulting from incomplete masculinization – clitoromegaly and urogenital sinus (Prader III–V degrees);

and the persistence of Mullerian structures (hypoplastic uterus, or rudimental uterine horns and Fallopian tubes).

Clinical Case. Young Patient A., 14 year old, with incomplewte 46,XY gonadal dysgenesis. (Fig. I-2a, b, c).

The external genitalia of this patient presented on Figure V-2 (Chappter V).

Figure I-2a. 46,XY gonadal dysgenesis with hypoplastic unicavital uterus, laparoscopy.

Testicle dysgenesis, Fallopian tubes, a normal shaped hypoplastic uterus and vagina.

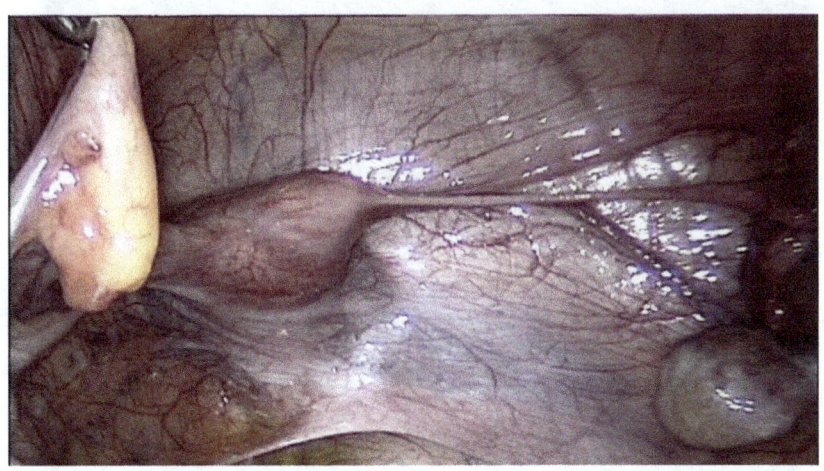

Figure I-2b. 46,XY gonadal dysgenesis.
Testicle dysgenesis with only Fallopian tube on the right side.

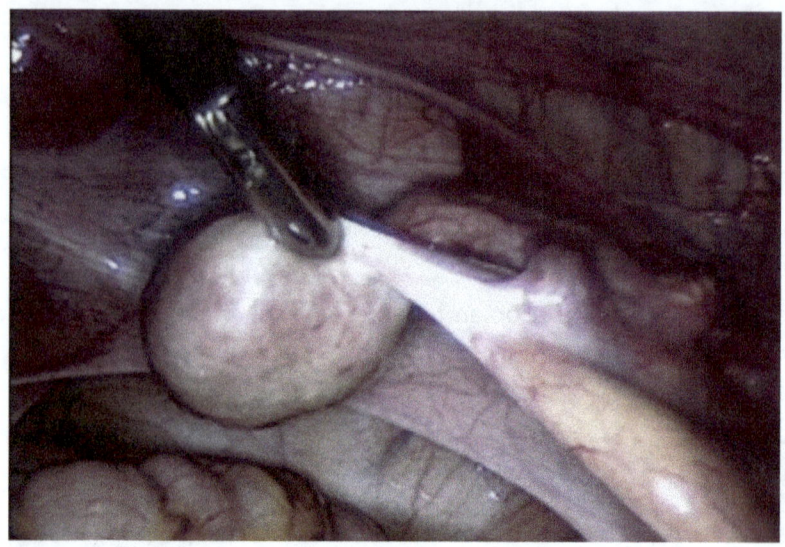

Figure I-2c. Testicular disgenesis, histology.

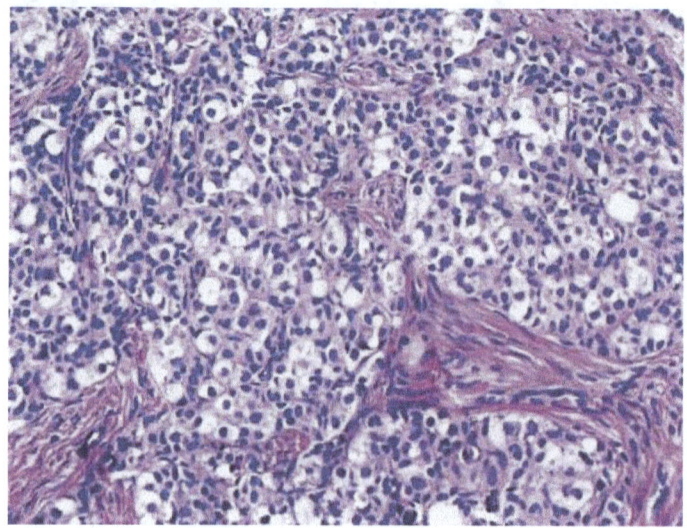

Adrenal insensitivity syndrome (AIS) is most commonly caused by mutations of the androgen receptor gene and may be either partial or complete. The testes of these individuals produce Mullerian inhibitory substance (MIS) and consequently the uterus, Fallopian tubes and vagina are absent. [15]

Patients with androgen insensitivity syndrome (AIS) exhibit testicular dysgenesis, which is histologically composed of small seminiferous tubules with a reduced diameter, immature Sertoli cells that are immature, lack a central lumen, and reach the Leydig cells.

In androgen insensitivity syndrome (AIS), depending on the residual activity of the androgen receptor, patients exhibit feminine external genitalia in a complete form, or ambiguous genitalia as a consequence of incomplete masculinization (in the incomplete form).

The ovotesticular gonads present with both testicular and ovarian tissues or as separate gonads. In the bilateral ovotestis, the testicular and ovarian components are adjacent to each other in an end-to-end manner.

Most ovotesticular DSD patients had a 46,XY karyotype, although some patients had a 46,XX karyotype or exhibited a Y-to X chromosomal translocation and chimerism (i.e., the presence of two or more cell lines derived from different zygotes).

A unique clinical case of ovotesticular DSD with rare form of chimerism was detected in a 1-year-old patient with a 46,XX/46,XY karyotype (Fig. I-3a, b, c). Both gonads presented as ovotestis in which the gonad on the left side (Fig. I-3-a) was associated with the Fallopian tube, while on the right side (Fig. I-3-b) it was associated with the ductus seminiferous alone. The persistent Mullerian ducts could be detected in the crossing area between the Fallopian tube (on the left) and ductus seminiferous (on the right) with gonadal ridges.

Figure I-3 (a, b). A unique clinical case of ovotesticular DSD with rare form of 46,XX/46,XY chimerism was detected in a 1-year-old patient. Laparoscopically, the both gonads were ambiguous.

Figure I-3a. The left ovotestis: predominated ovarian (O) tissue (yellow), with whitish testicular structure on the upper pole, associated with the Fallopian tube (F) only.

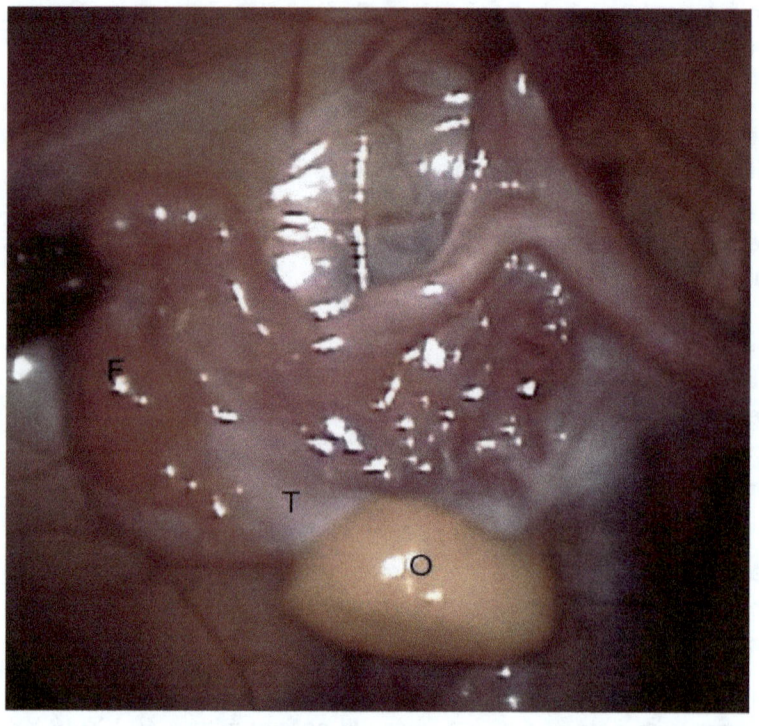

Figure I-3b. The right ovotestis: predominated testicular tissue (T), with small ovarian structure (yellow) on the upper pole (O), associated with the ductus seminiferous (DS) alone.

The ovarian (O) part seems like appendix testis.

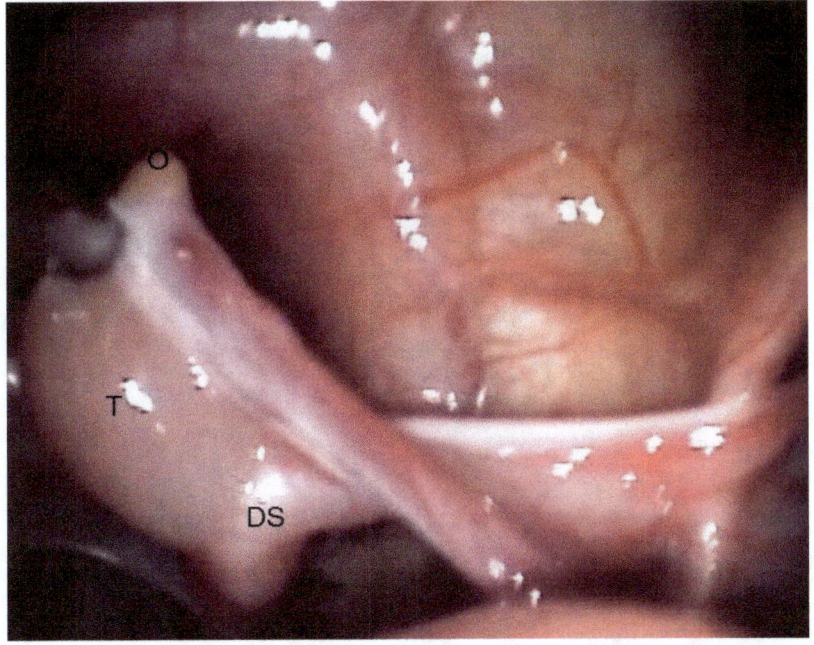

Figure I-3c. Ovotesticular DSD. Prader stage III.

Clitoromegaly and sinus urogenitalis resulted of incomplete posterior labial fusion.

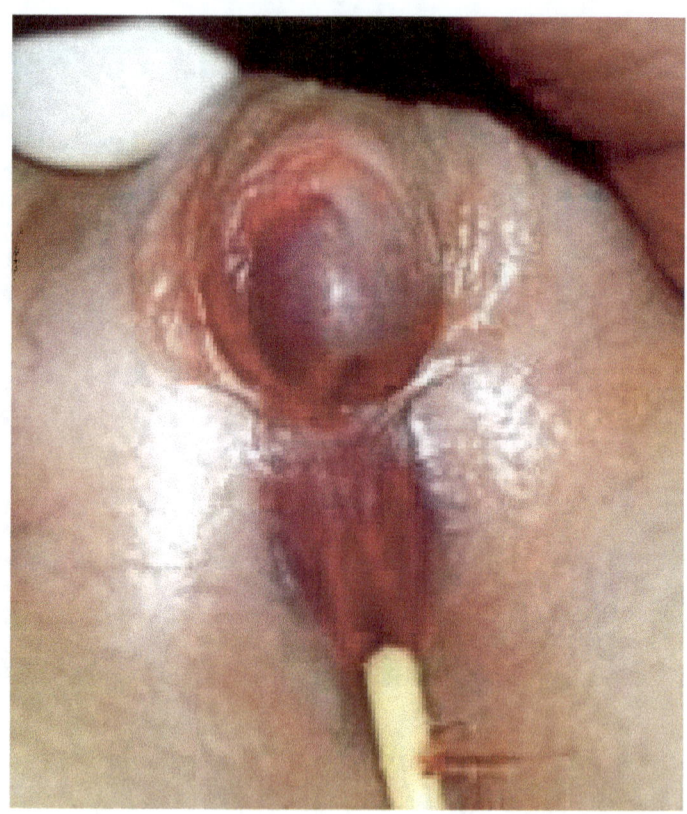

Figure I-3d. Ovotestis. The ovarian component on the left and the testicular parenchyma on the right side.

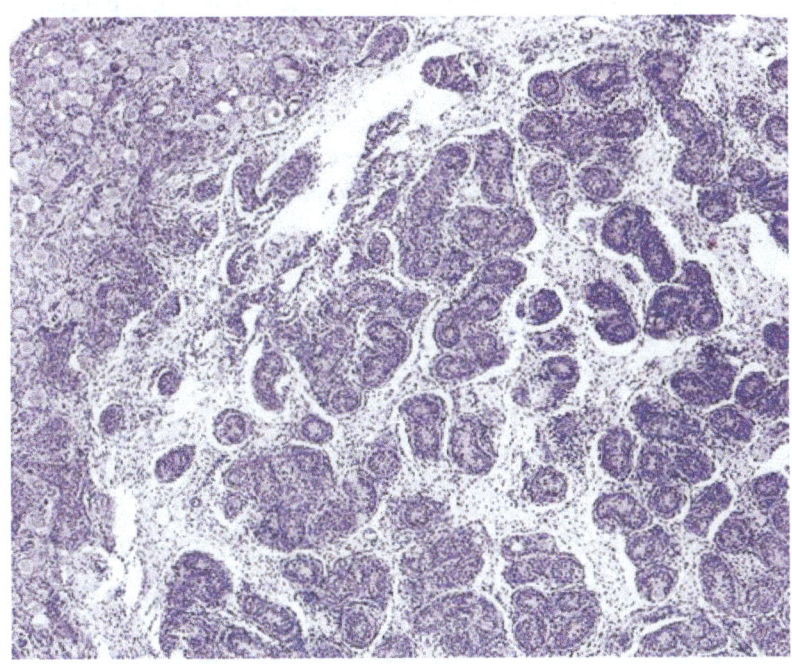

Persistent Mullerian duct syndrome (PMDS) is a rare form of DSD, in which Mullerian ducts derivatives occur in genotypic 46,XY patients (Fig. I-2). The internal genitalia in PMDS patients presents as uterine rudiments or hypoplastic uterine horns and Fallopian tubes. The uterine rudiments in all cases could be detected in the crossing area of the Fallopian tubes with gonadal ridges. The external genitalia were ambiguous because of variable degrees of virilization.

PMDS may result from Sertoli cell-specific dysfunction resulting from mutations in the MIS gene with normal fetal Leydig and Sertoli cell function.

Defective androgen action is associated with female or ambiguous genitalia.

Importantly, in PMDS patients with a 46,XY karyotype and testicular gonads, the Fallopian tubes or ductus deferens persisted separately on the unilateral or bilateral sides. In none of these cases did both types of ducts persist on either side.

Based on these findings, we propose a novel hypothesis which predicts that the Fallopian tubes, similarly to the seminiferous ducts, are analogous and develop from mesonephric ducts.

Conclusions

Systematic clinical analysis and a literature review revealed the following controversies and questions:

- What is the embryonal pathogenesis of ambiguous gonads - ovotestis?
- Why do most ovotesticular patients have a 46,XY karyotype?
- Why do SRY-negative ovotesticular patients with a 46,XX karyotype have testicular components in their gonads?
- In 46,XX-male syndrome, why do the SRY-negative patients have testes?
- How do some 46,XY DSD patients develop Mullerian ducts derivatives, including Fallopian tubes, uterine rudiments or a hypoplastic uterus and vagina?

A new hypothesis to describe gonadal embryogenesis

The indifferent gonad (Fig. I-4a) is differentiating into an ovary (Fig. I-4b) or testis (Fig. I-4c) because of its chromosomal sex, which is either 46,XX (SRY-negative) or 46,XY (SRY-positive), respectively.

Male or female pathways of gonadal development are different, but share some common features.

Male gonadal development (testis) (Fig. I-4c)
The primitive sex cords are proliferating and penetrate deep into the gonadal medulla to form the lobuli of the testis.
The major determinative factor for the testes is SRY-dependent influences of the mesonephric system (mesonephric tubules and corpuscles) on gonadal masculinization. Mesonephric derivatives persist and form the main genital ducts of the male embryo. Excretory tubules of the mesonephric system form the seminiferous tubules, which join to the rete testis and develop into the ductuli deferentes. Sustentacular cells of Sertoli are derived from the mesonephric excretory tubules. The interstitial Leydig cells are derived from the original mesenchyme of the mesonephros. The mesonephric tubules have inductive influences on the primordial gonads (germ cells) to drive the development of the indifferent gonad into testis. If the mesonephric tubules recede, the gonads will not differentiate and the indifferent gonads will remain as an ovary.

Female gonadal development (ovary) (Fig. I-4b)
In contrast to the most prevalent current opinion, the original mesonephric cells (tubules and corpuscles) persist in the ovarian parenchyma.
In the female gonads, some mesonephric excretory tubules recede and then lose their tubular structure; however, most of them persist and form ovarian theca interna and externa. The theca interna and externa support the processes of oocyte proliferation, maturity and ovulation, similarly to the Sertoli cells in the male gonads.

Hence, ovarian theca interna and externa are analogous to the sustentacular Sertoli cells in the testis. The interstitial Leydig cells in the ovary are derived from the intertubal mesenchyme of the mesonephros, similar to the male gonad (testis). Reduction of the mesonephric tubular system in the gonads results in female gonadal development. After regression of mesonephric tubules occurs, the mesonephric ducts persist and develop into Fallopian tubes with cranial opening of fimbrial orifice.

According to the new hypothesis, the Fallopian tubes and seminiferous ducts are analogues, as they both develop from the mesonephric ducts (in female or male embryos, respectively), which can account for the etiology of persistent Mullerian ducts derivate in 46,XY DSD patients (Table I-1, Fig. I-4).

The uterus (uterine fold) develops near the intersection between the mesonephral ducts and the gonadal ridge.

The major determinative factor in the sexual differentiation of gonads is the mesonephros, represented by the embryonic kidney (provisory urinary system). The excretory ducts of both males (ductus deferens) and females (Fallopian tubes) develop from the mesonephric ducts.

The ovotestis forms during the intermediate stage of normal testis embryogenesis, while the gonads presented with both testicular and ovarian tissue.

Alfred Jost showed that testicular organization is marked by the development of pre-Sertoli cells, which progressively surround germ cells to form seminiferous tubules in the testes only.418

Ditewig, Yao (2005) consider the process of ovary organogenesis as the default organ, which develops in the absence of testis-promoting factors. Bisexual development of the gonads is a universal phenomenon in vertebrates.19

Based on our new hypothesis, the interstitial Leydig cells can differentiate into both gonads (testis and ovary) from the intertubal mesenchyme of the mesonephros.

The cranial tubules and glomeruli of the mesonephros degenerate and partially disappear. In the intermediate stage, the gonad exhibits bipotential: the cranial part of the indifferent gonad becomes ovarian after regression of the mesonephric tubules, while in the caudal part the mesonephric ducts persist and participate in forming the testicular tissue.

Consequently, the ovotestis progresses into the intermediate stage of normal testis embryogenesis, in which the gonads are present with both testicular and ovarian tissue.

By contrast, most ovotesticular DSD patients have a 46,XY karyotype (or SRY-positive).

While most mesonephric tubules reduced, the mesonephric ducts become the Fallopian tubes. The excretory ducts of both males and females develop from mesonephric ducts. Therefore, the Fallopian tubes and seminiferous ducts can be considered to be analogues, and both develop from the mesonephric ducts (in female or male embryos, respectively), which could explain the phenomenon of Mullerian duct persistence in genetically 46,XY patients who have testicular dysgenesis.

Over 150 cases have been reported in which SRY-negative 46,XX testicular DSD patients present with small testes and androgen deficiency, and in some cases with ambiguous genitalia. [12, 13, 15]

Surprisingly, the leading determinative factor in sexual differentiation of the gonads is the mesonephros, represented by the embryonic kidney (urinary system).

Embryogenesis in the human urogenital system is intimately interwoven with sex differentiation. Proliferation of the mesonephric system (tubules and corpuscles) in the gonads stimulates masculinization of the gonads into testis. Reduction of the mesonephric tubular system in the gonads results in female gonad development.

The intermediate locus between the gonadal ridge and mesonephros becomes the mesosalpyngs in female embryos. The paraovarian cysts in mesosalpyngs are derived from mesonephric tubules.

The vestigial structures after regression of mesonephros are persisting in embryo. Probably, the epoophoron and paroophoron are remnant of a few scattered rudimentary mesonephric tubules situated in the mesosalpings in females. The regressed upper pole of gonadal ridge with mesonephric tubules in male embryo may become the rudimental appendix testis (Fig. I-3b).

If we accept a mesonephric origin of the Fallopian tubes, we can account for the determinative influence of the Fallopian tubes in the ovarian cancer.

Future embryological studies of sex differentiation will of great importance to test the applicability of this new hypothesis.

Figure I-4. Gonadal Sex Differentiation: A new hypothesis.

Schematic representation of gonadal differentiation from the genital ridge (GR – blue), mesonephros (Ms – red), and mesonephric duct (MD – red).

Fig. I-4a. The indifferent gonad and mesonephros.

The gonadal ridge (GR-blue) grows longitudinally. The paramedial side the gonad connects with the mesonephros (Ms). The mesonephric tubules progressively surround the germ cells in gonadal ridge to form the Sertoli cells.

The cranial tubules and glomeruli of the mesonephros (dashed horizontal red lines)degenerate and partially disappear. The cranial part of the indifferent gonad becomes ovarian after regression of the mesonephric tubules.

In the caudal section, the mesonephric ducts persist (solid horizontal red lines) and participate in the formation of testicular tissue (ductuli semynipherous, rete testis and ductuli efferentes).

The mesonephric duct (MD) grows on the lateral side of the mesonephros (Ms), then crosses medially to the gonadal ridge. The area of intersection between the mesonephric duct and the gonadal ridge develops into the uterine fold (U) in females and the prostatic utricle in males.

The intermediate stage of gonadal differentiation consists of ovarian (Ov) and testicular (T) tissue, which corresponds to ovotestis.

Fig. I-4b. Female gonad differentiation: SRY-negative, ovary.

In the female gonads, germ cells (from gonadal ridge) become oocytes and granulosa cells. Some mesonephric excretory tubules regress, and some lose their tubular structure, but most persist as Sertoli cells and form theca interna and externa, which surround oocytes in primordial follicles. In the female embryo, the upper part of the gonadal ridge (before intersecting with the mesonephric ducts) form ovary and ligamentum ovary; the lower part represents the ligamentum teres uteri.

While most mesonephric tubules recede, the mesonephric ducts (MD) become Fallopian tubes.

Fig. I-4c. Male gonad differentiation: SRY-positive, testis.

In the male gonads, germ cells become spermatozoids. Mesonephric tubules surround the germ cells in the ductus seminiferous and form Sertoli cells. While most mesonephric tubules persist, the mesonephric ducts become ductus deferens. The Leydig cells are derived from mesonephric intertubular mesenchyme in both gonads.

The Fallopian tubes (in females) and the seminiferous duct (in males) are analogous, and both develop from the mesonephral ducts.

Figure I-4. Gonadal Sex Differentiation: A new hypothesis.

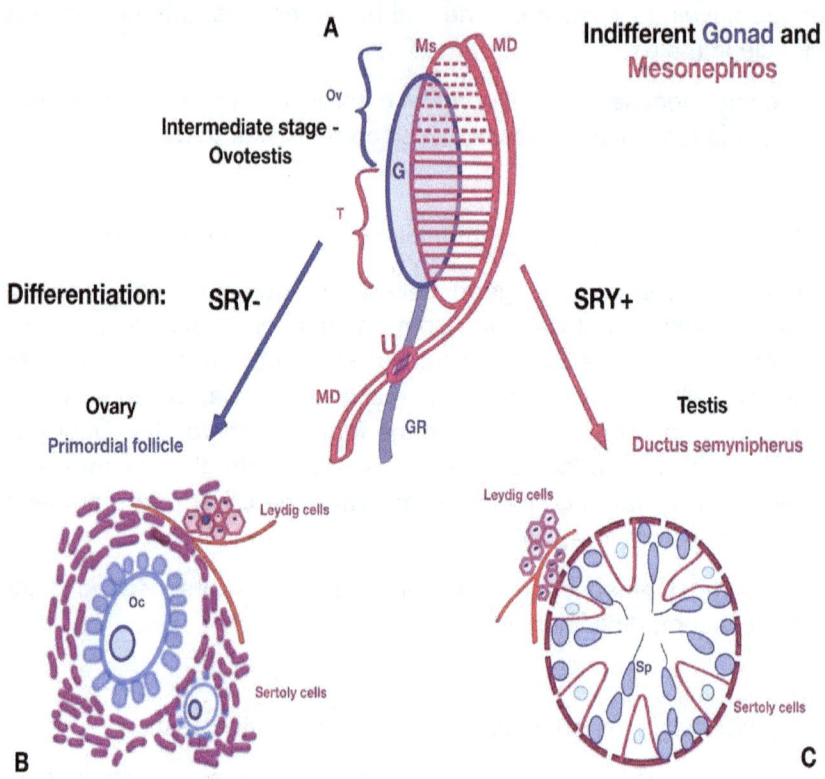

Tab. I-1. Gonadal differentiation: key differences between the new hypothesis and contemporary view.

	New Hypothesis		Contemporary View [1–6]	
	Testis	Ovary	Testis	Ovary
Embryonal derivates				
germ cells	spermatozoids	oocytes, granulosa cells	spermatozoids	oocytes
mesonephric tubules	sustentacular Sertoly cells	theca interna and externa	sustentacular Sertoly cells	reduces
intertubal mesenchyme of mesonephros	interstitial Leydig cells	interstitial Leydig cells	reduces	reduces
mesonephric ducts	ductus deferens, rete testis	Fallopian tubes and vagina. Uterus forms in crossing area between mesonephric ducts with genital ridges	ductus deferens, rete testis	reduces
mesenchyme of the genital ridge	tunica albuginea and lobuli of testis	tunica albuginea	interstitial Leydig cells	interstitial Leydig cells

References

1. Sadler TW. "Langman`s Medical Embryology". IX-th edn, Baltimore:Lippincott Williams&Wilkins, 2000, 230-256.
2. Sadler TW. "Langman`s Medical Embryology". XII-th edn, Baltimore:Lippincott Williams&Wilkins, 2012; 232-259
3. Hill MA. (2014) Embryology BGD Lecture - Sexual Differentiation. Retrieved October 16, 2014. Available from URL: http://php.med.unsw.edu.au/embryology/index.php?title=BGD_Lecture_Sexual_Differentiation
4. Jost A. A new look at the mechanism controlling sex differentiation in mammals. Johns Hopkins Med J 1972;130:28-36.
5. Hughes IA, Houk C, Ahmed SF, et al. Consensus statement on management of intersex disorders. Archives of Disease in Childhood, 2006; 91, 554–563. doi.org/10.1136/adc.2006.098319
6. Brain CE, Creighton SM, Mushtaq I. et al. Holistic management of DSD. Best Practice and Research. Clinical Endocrinology and Metabolism, 2010; 24, 335–354.
7. Pasterski V, Prentice P, Hughes IA. Consequences of the Chicago consensus on disorders of sex development (DSD): current practices in Europe. Archives of Disease in Childhood, 2010; 95, 618–623. doi:10.1136/adc.2009.163840
8. Houk CP, Lee PA. Update on disorders of sex development. Curr Opin Endocrinol Diabetes Obes, 2012; 19:28-32. doi: 10.1097/MED.0b013e32834edacb
9. Ahmed F, Achermann J, Arlt W, et al. UK guidance on the initial evaluation of an infant or an adolescent with a suspected disorder of sex development. Clin Endocrinol (Oxf). 2011 July; 75(1): 12–26. doi: 10.1111/j.1365-2265.2011.04076.x
10. Achermann JC, Hughes IA, Disorders of sex development. In: Kronenberg HM, Melmed S, Polonsky KS, Larsen PR (eds) Williams Textbook of Endocrinology 11th edition, Philadelphia; 2008, 783-848.
11. Cools, M., Nordenström, A., Robeva, R. et al. Caring for individuals with a difference of sex development (DSD): a Consensus

Statement. Nat Rev Endocrinol 14, 415–429 (2018). https://doi.org/10.1038/s41574-018-0010-8.

12. Chemes H, Muzulin PM, Venara MC, Mulhmann M del C, Martinez M, Gamboni M. Early manifestations of testicular dysgenesis in children: pathological phenotypes, karyotype correlations and precursor stages of tumor development. APMIS. 2003;111(1):12-23. doi:10.1034/j.1600-0463.2003.1110104.x

13. Nistal M, García-Fernández E, Mariño-Enríquez A. et al. Usefulness of gonadal biopsy in the diagnosis of sexual developmental disorders. Actas Urol Esp 2007;31:9:1056-1075.

14. Prader A, Gartner HP. The syndrome of male pseudohermaphroditism in adrenocortical hyperplasia without overproduction of androgens. Helv Pediatric Acta 1955;10:397-412.

15. Nathalie Josso, Rodolfo Rey, Jean-Yves Picard. Testicular Anti-Müllerian Hormone: Clinical Applications in DSD. Semin Reprod Med 2012; 30(05): 364-373 doi: 10.1055/s-0032-1324719

16. Thyen U, Lanz K, Holterhus PM, Hiort O. Epidemiology and initial management of ambiguous genitalia at birth in Germany. Horm Res 2006, 66(4):195-203. doi:10.1159/000094782

17. Bernard Crespi. Turner syndrome and the evolution of human sexual dimorphism Evol Appl. 2008 August; 1(3): 449–461. doi: 10.1111/j.1752-4571.2008.00017.x

18. Josso N. Professor Alfred Jost: the builder of modern sex differentiation. Sex Dev. 2008;2(2):55-63. doi: 10.1159/000129690. Epub 2008 Jun 20.

19. Ditewig AC, Yao HH. Organogenesis of the ovary: a comparative review on vertebrate ovary formation. Organogenesis. 2005 Apr;2(2):36-41. doi:10.4161/org.2.2.2491

II. UTEROVAGINAL ANATOMIC DEVIATIONS

Introduction

Organogenesis of the human female reproductive tract is a complex, multistage process from the initial ambisexual stage to final morphogenesis. Congenital or structural variations can arise during abnormal embryonal development (Isaacson et al., 2018; Cunha et al., 2018). Most congenital variations can be identified prenatally or at birth (also known as birth defects), but some may only be detected later in infancy or even in adult life (World Health Organization, 2018).

Major structural or genetic birth defects affect approximately 3-4% of newborns, and account for 20% of all infant mortality (Monlleo et al., 2012; Matthews et al., 2015; European Surveillance of Congenital Anomalies (EUROCAT), 2017). Among all congenital anomalies, the estimated prevalence of genital malformations is 12% (Hill, 2020), and these malformations are third in frequency after heart and limb defects (EUROCAT, 2017).

A systemic review by Chan et al. (2011) revealed that the incidence of uterovaginal variations in adult females is 5.5% in the general population, but it is higher in infertile women (8%) and women with pregnancy loss (13.3%). An arcuate uterus was reportedly the most common anomaly in an unselected population (3.9%), and a septate uterus was the most frequent anomaly in high-risk populations (Chan et al., 2011; Cunha et al., 2018). According to Dietrich et al. (2014) and Prior et al. (2018), clinical examination of newborns usually includes only an inspection of external genitalia. Therefore, few female genital abnormalities are correctly identified at birth, and most cases are under-reported or diagnosed later in adult life.

For example, most patients with complete or partial vaginal aplasia and a functional rudimentary horn are diagnosed at menarche or later, due to severe abdominal pain, peritoneal symptoms, and menstrual outflow obstruction or retrograde flow (Dietrich et al., 2014). A report by Paradisi et al. (2014) estimated that 24.5% of infertile women with a history of miscarriage have congenital uterine variations; these may be diagnosed and corrected too late to prevent complications. Only 25-37% of patients with uterovaginal variations have successful reproductive outcomes, despite minimally invasive surgical correction and assisted reproductive methods.

The clinical manifestations and surgical treatment of structural variations depend on the variant anatomy. Hence, anatomic classification has a primary role in the verification of the type of anomaly and is necessary for appropriate surgery and management (Buttram and Gibbons, 1979; Grimbizis et al., 2013; Heinonen, 2016; Acien et al., 2016a). However, many anatomic variations do not align well with currently available classification systems. Therefore, a new classification system based on embryological development stages is proposed to facilitate diagnosis and treatment for patients with uterovaginal variations.

Materials and methods

Medical records were reviewed for surgical treatments of 1320 patients with various uterovaginal variations between 1998 and 2022 at the National Medical Research Center for Obstetrics, Gynecology, and Perinatology in Moscow, Russia.

The anatomic types of uterovaginal variations were diagnosed by 3D ultrasound or magnetic resonance imaging (MRI), and then verified by laparoscopy. Reconstructive surgery was performed in accordance with variant anatomy, patient's symptoms, concomitant pathology, and complications. After clinical examination of females with various forms of DSD, karyotyping, studies of gonadal morphology, and hormonal measurements were conducted. All cases were categorized using a new anatomic classification system based on embryonic developmental stages.

All patients signed informed consent for surgical procedures; if adolescent patients were under 18, the written informed consent was obtained from a parent. Informed consent for the study was not required due to the retrospective design.

Results

Uterovaginal variations (deviations) were grouped according to 11 types and 24 anatomic variants and described according to their clinical presentations and morphological patterns (Variants 1-8). The new Anatomic Classification of Uterovaginal Variants is presented in Figure II-1. The clinical management and appropriate surgical treatment proposed according to the defined anatomic variations are summarized in Table II-1.

Patient classifications and treatments

Type 1. Uterovaginal aplasia

Definition: an aplastic uterus and vagina, with either non-functional (variant 1a) or functional (variant 1b) rudiments.

Variant 1a: Uterovaginal aplasia with non-functional rudiments

Uterine and vaginal aplasia (Mayer-Rokitansky-Kuster-Hauser syndrome) are thought to correspond to the earliest stage of embryonal development. Patients with uterovaginal aplasia had a normal 46,XX karyotype, but 10% had 45,X/46,XX mosaicism and ovarian dysgenesis (a mosaic variant of Turner syndrome). All Type patients had uterine rudiments, with normally-shaped fallopian tubes and ovaries. Most had slender myometrial cords in the area of intersection between the fallopian tubes and round (broad) and ovarian ligaments, which qualified as nonfunctional uterine rudiments without endometrial cavities (Variant 1a).

Surgery: creation of a neovagina with removal of the uterine rudiments in patients with pelvic pain and endometriosis.

Variant 1a: Uterovaginal aplasia with non-functional rudiments

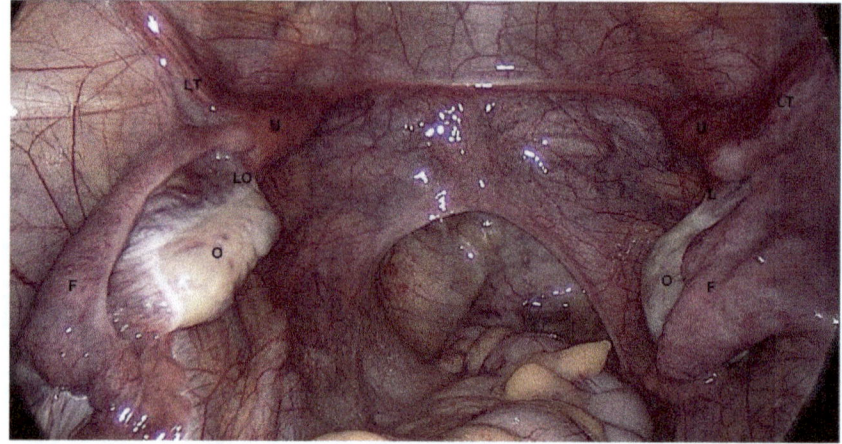

Variant 1b: Uterovaginal aplasia with functional rudiments

Some patients with uterovaginal aplasia had uterine rudiments (horns) with functional endometrial cavities in the area of intersection between the fallopian tubes and round (broad), and ovarian ligaments.

Laparoscopy in young patients with periodic abdominal pain revealed retrograde menstrual outflow from the functional rudiments into the peritoneal cavity.

Surgery: removal of functional uterine rudiments with creation of a neovagina.

Variant 1b Uterovaginal aplasia, functional rudiments.

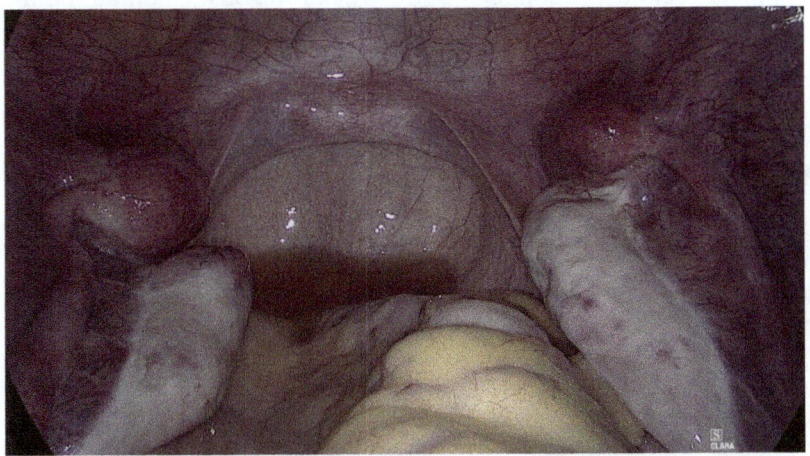

Type 2. Cervicovaginal aplasia

Definition: a functional unicavital uterus, with an aplastic cervix and vagina. Variants 2a and 2b depend on the degree of cervical and vaginal development.

Complete vaginal aplasia was usually combined with cervical maldevelopment; the uterus was normally shaped, with a blind endometrial cavity. This anomaly was typically diagnosed in adolescent females at the time of menarche due to menstrual outflow obstruction. The uterine cavity was small and non-extensible; retrograde menstrual bleeding caused severe acute abdominal pain with intense peritoneal symptoms due to hematometra, hematosalpinx, or hemoperitoneum. MRI was preferred to distinguish the 2 anatomical subtypes (variants) of cervicovaginal aplasia, which required different surgical treatment.

Variant 2a: rudimentary unicavital uterus with complete cervical agenesis and vaginal aplasia

Variant 2a: Laparoscopic view – normally shaped uterus with complete cervical agenesis and vaginal aplasia, hematometra, hemoperytoneum.

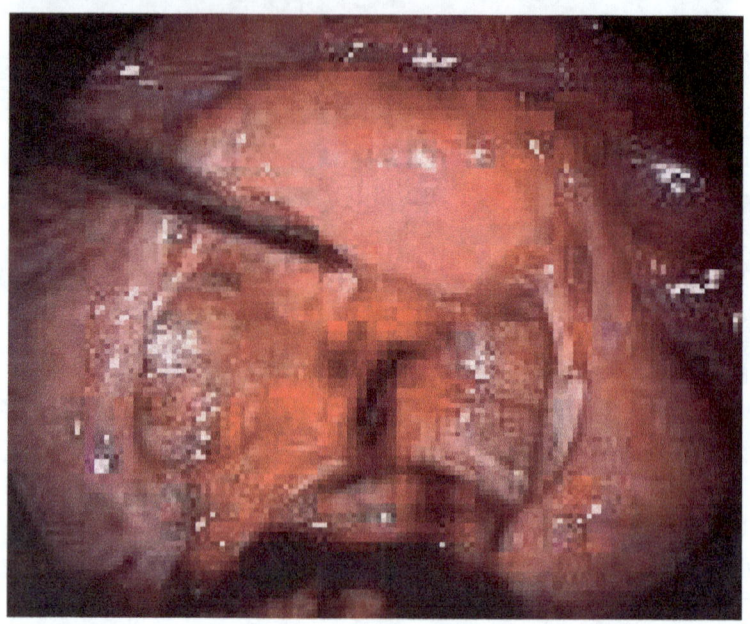

Variant 2b: unicavital uterus and cervical aplasia, with a blind cervix and absence of a cervical canal
Surgery: laparoscopic drainage and evacuation of hemorrhagic liquid from the uterine tubes and peritoneal cavity; uterovaginal or uteroperitoneal stenting (or uterovaginal anastomosis), with sparing of the functional uterus.

These uterine variations are categorized as having the most difficult reconstructive surgery. New methods of uterine preservation are being developed.

In cases of rudimentary uterus with cervical agenesis (Variant II-2-a), uterine preservation is ineffective, because secondary atresia has occurred in most cases. Histological investigation reveals deep myometrial dystrophy accompanying the severe anatomical defect.

The creation of a neovagina from a peritoneal pouch is possible (Acien et al., 2016b; Rezaei et al., 2016). In inoperable cases, trans-myometrial embryo transfer may be considered.

Variant 2b: unicavital uterus and cervical aplasia, with a blind cervix and absence of a cervical canal

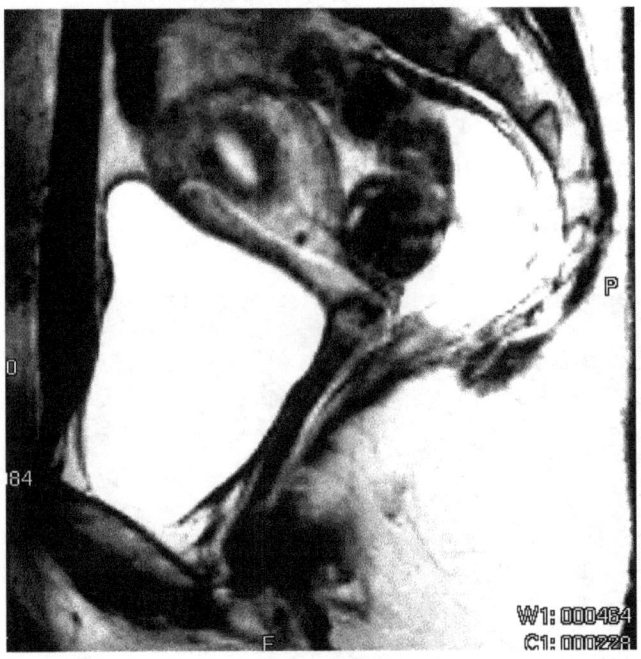

Type 3. Partial vaginal aplasia
Definition: normal uterus with partially aplastic vagina.
Variant 3a: Partial vaginal aplasia
Congenital deficiency of vaginal growth and connection to the vulva (vestibulum vaginae) results in partial aplasia of the distal 2/3 or 1/3 of the vagina, with respective increases in distance between the vaginal pole and vestibulum vaginae. The entrance to the vagina is absent. While this may be diagnosed in newborns or adolescent

females with vaginoscopy, in most of the cases reviewed it was revealed during puberty due to severe pain, caused by menstrual outflow obstruction. Adolescent females experienced cyclic pain starting with menarche, made worse by overflow from the blind vagina. These patients usually presented to the hospital after 2-3 menstrual cycles, and were found to have hematocolpos, hematometra, hematosalpinx, or hemoperitoneum.
Surgery: vaginoplasty with laparoscopy for drainage and evacuation of hemorrhagic liquid from the uterine tubes and peritoneal cavity.

Variant 3a: MRI – partial (distal 1/3) vaginal aplasia, hematocolpos, hematometra.

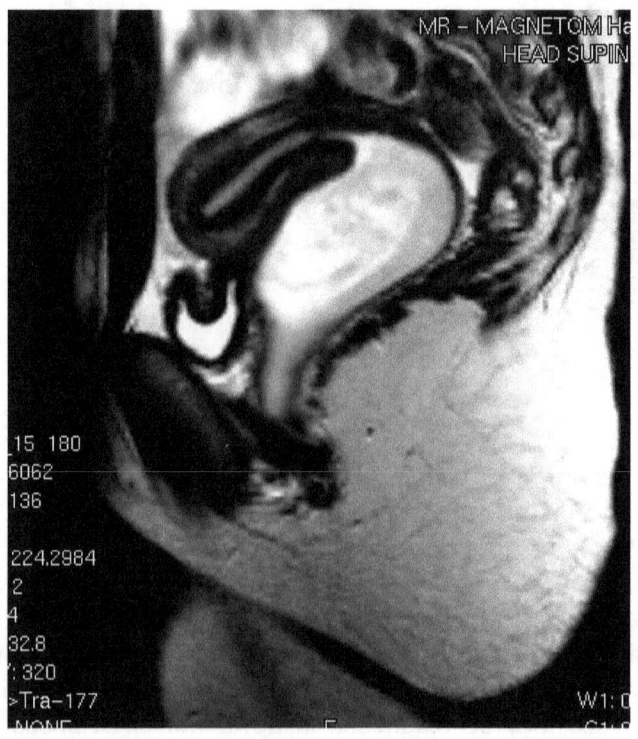

Variant 3b: Hymen imperforatum

Definition: a normal unicavital uterus; a normal vagina with a blind ending and an unperforated hymenal membrane.

A hymenal septum at the vaginal introitus is connected to the vestibulum and perforates due to physiological apoptosis. Imperforate hymen may be diagnosed in newborn females, due to mucous discharge obstruction (mucocolpos).

Surgery: a circular incision; laparoscopy in cases with hematocolpos and hematometra.

Variant 3b: MRI - hymen imperforatum, severe hematocolpos.

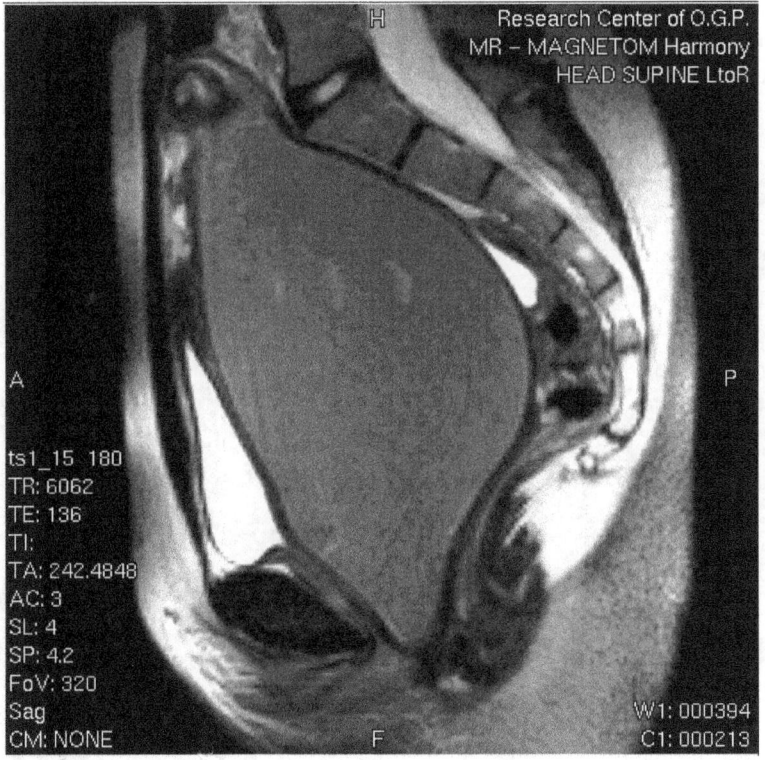

Type 4. Double uterus and vagina

Definition: a duplicated uterine corpus forming two hemiuteri, which connect separately to a duplicated cervix; duplicate vagina.

Variant 4a: Double uterus with complete or incomplete doubling of the vagina (symmetric form)

Surgery and management: resection of the longitudinal vaginal septum; functional MRI to determine which hemiuterus has better blood perfusion for embryo transfer in an in vitro fertilization (IVF) program.

Variant 4a: Laparoscopic view - double uterus (symmetric form), extragenital endometriosis.

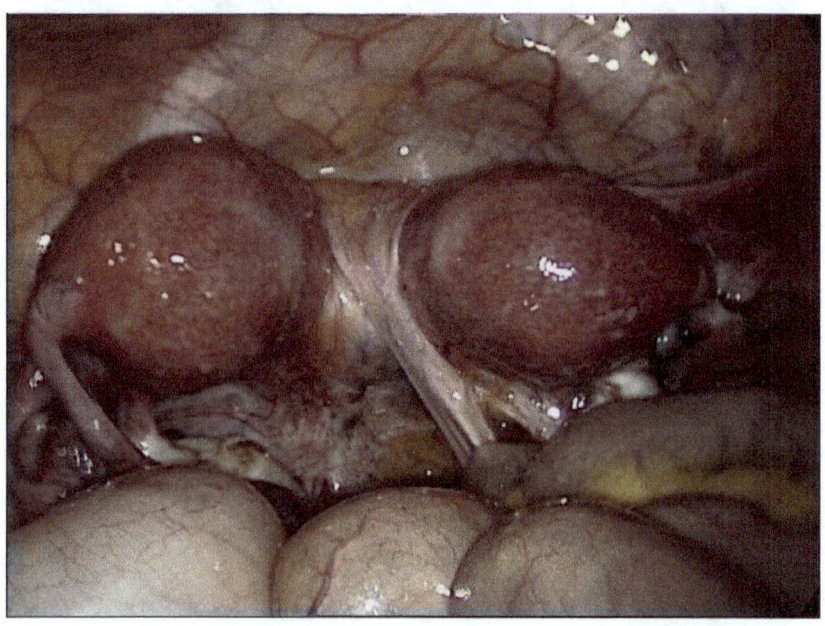

Variant 4a: completely doubling vagina (symmetric form).

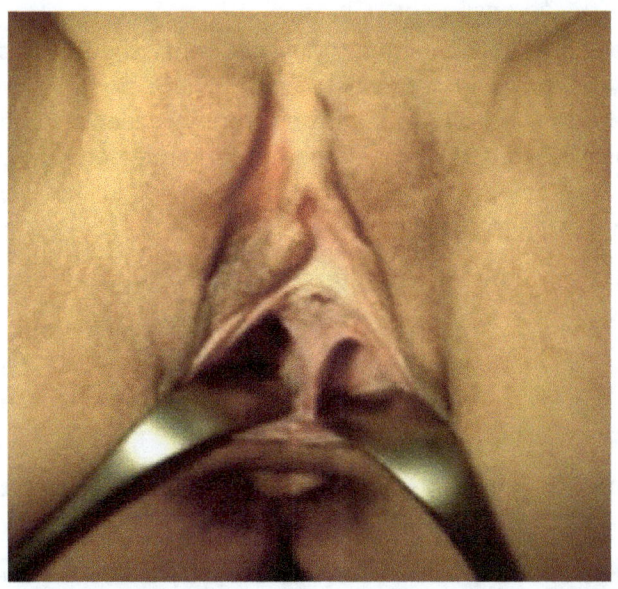

Variant 4b: Double uterus and vagina with partial aplasia of the hemivagina (asymmetric form)

Surgery: resection of the common longitudinal septum to restore menstrual outflow; laparoscopy for evacuation of retrograde menstrual flow.

Type 5. Completely septate uterus

Definition: an externally normal uterus with a complete intrauterine septum creating two endometrial cavities and cervical canals and a divided cervix. The vagina may be duplicated or normal.

A completely septate uterus develops by fusion of the two hemiuteri. Successful pregnancy without metroplasty has been found to be possible in 46% of these cases, depending on vascularization of the septum. However, in 54% of patients, microcirculation in the complete intrauterine septum was found to be reduced to 22-35% of that in the myometrium, resulting in a need for resection of the septum (Makiyan et al., 2016). Functional (DCE) MRI is required for estimation of blood perfusion in the complete septum in non-pregnant (or infertile) patients. Operative treatment is preferred when blood perfusion is reduced by ≥20% in the septum as compared to the myometrium, or in those with a history of miscarriage (Makiyan et al., 2016).

Variant 5a: Complete septate uterus, double cervix and vagina

Surgery: resection of the longitudinal vaginal septum, then estimation of the distance between the cervical canals. When the length is ≥ 6 mm, hysteroresectoscopy is performed between the internal cervical ostium and fundal level.

Variant 5a: MRI - completely septate uterus, doubling cervix and cervical canal.

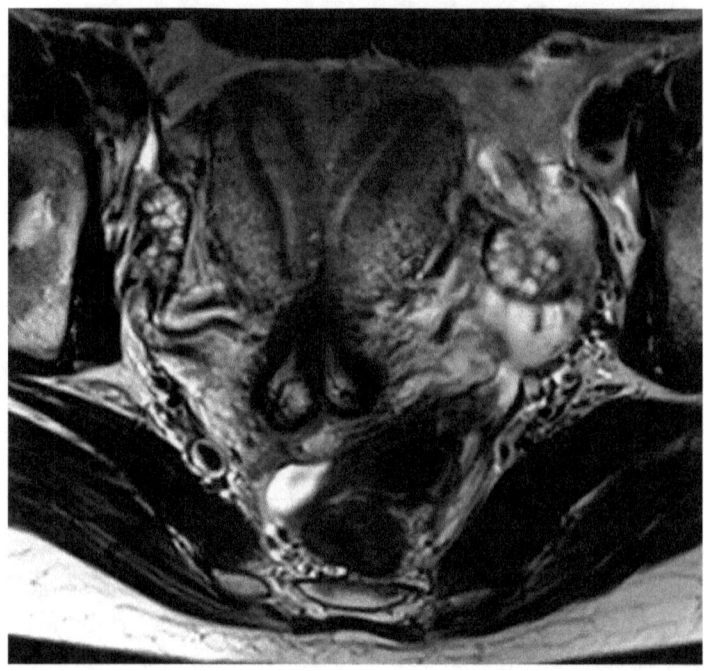

Variant 5a. Complete intrauterine septum. Successful pregnancy without metroplasty. Cesarean section performed, the newborn located in the left hemiutery.

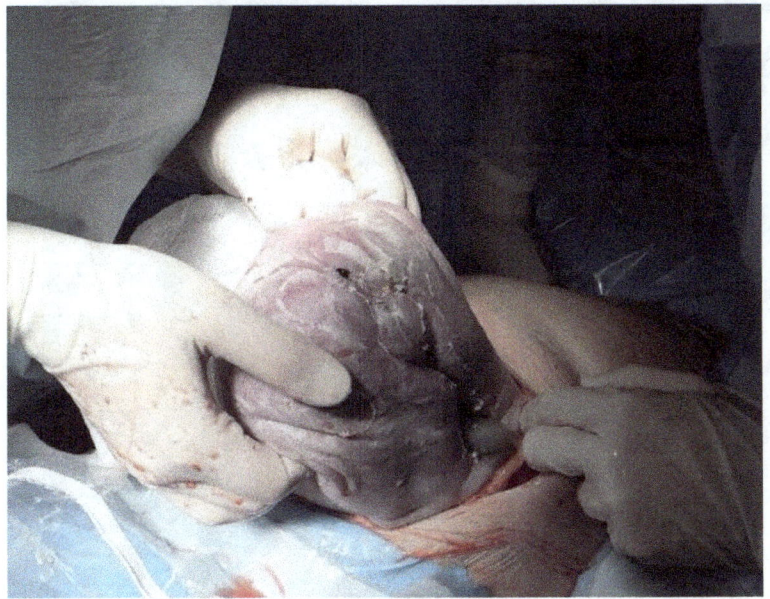

Complete intrauterine septum.

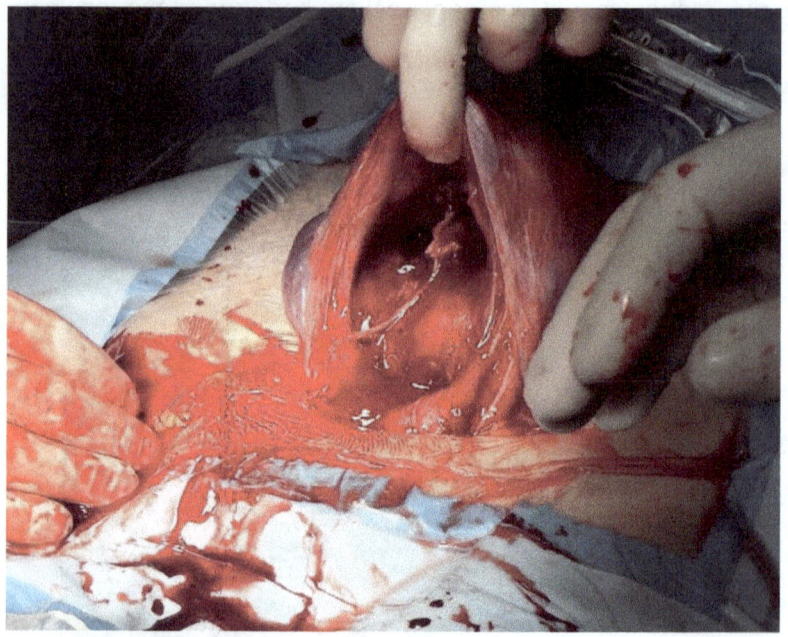

The uterus has normally shaped outline.

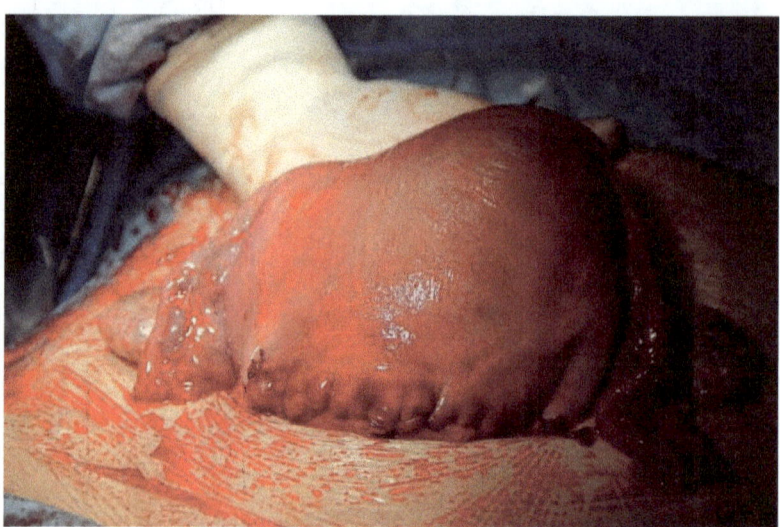

Variant 5b: Complete septate uterus and cervical canal, double vagina

Surgery: resection of the longitudinal vaginal septum. When the common cervix length is ≤6 mm, and the cervical canal is doubled, complete hysteroresectoscopy is performed for the creation of a unicavital uterus and cervical canal.

Variant 5c: Complete septate uterus and double vagina with partial aplasia of the hemivagina (asymmetric form, as in Variant 4b).

Surgery: resection of the common longitudinal septum to restore menstrual outflow; laparoscopy for evacuation of retrograde menstrual flow.

Type 6. Bicornuate uterus

Definition: a symmetric bicornuate uterus (two-horned), with both hemiuteri fused together and conjoined to a single cervix with a common cervical canal; normal vagina. Complete (**Variant 6a**) and incomplete (**Variant 6b**) forms of bicornuate uterus are recognized.

The incomplete bicornuate uterus (Variant 6b) may be confused with another variation – incomplete uterine septum (Type 8). In addition, an asymmetric bicornuate uterus with a non-communicating unilateral rudimentary horn is similar to a unicornuate uterus with a rudimentary horn (Type 7). It is important to distinguish these bicornuate variants from other Types, as the surgical approaches differ.

Surgery: reconstructive surgery is not necessary, because the reproductive prognosis is optimistic due to adequate blood perfusion in the bicornuate uterus.

Type 6. Laparoscopic view - bicornuate uterus

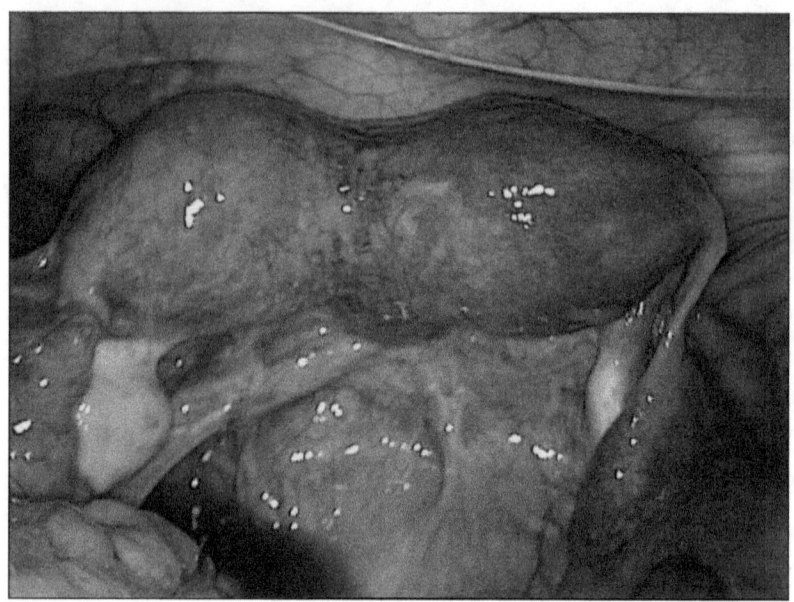

Type 7. Unicornuate uterus

Definition: an asymmetric unicornuate (one-horned) uterus conjoined to a single cervix with a common cervical canal; normal vagina. The second horn is rudimentary, and four Variants are recognized.

This Type is distinct from a unicornuate uterus with a communicating rudimentary horn, which is considered bicornuate, even if asymmetric.

Variant 7a: Unicornuate uterus with rudimentary horn with functional endometrial cavity
The functional rudimentary horn with an endometrial cavity is always detected in the crossing area between the fallopian tubes with ovarian and broad ligaments.

Variant 7a: Laparoscopy - unicornuate uterus with rudimentary functional horn. There is a heterotopic pregnancy in the right rudimentary horn. The rudimentary horn removed.

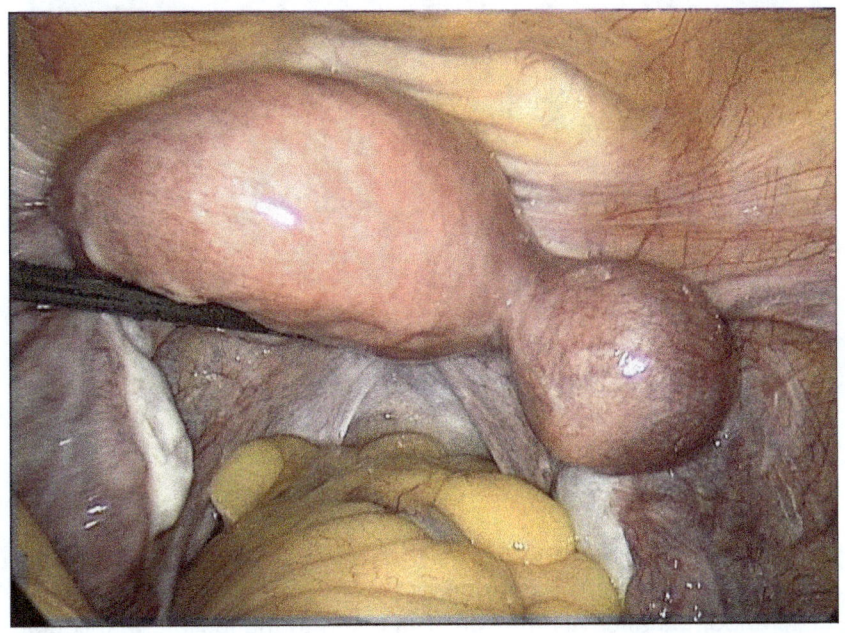

Variant 7b: Unicornuate uterus with rudimentary non-functional horn
Although the horn is nonfunctional, eutopic endometrial glands in the horn may grow and disseminate, causing ectopic endometriosis in the uterine mass.

Variant 7b: Unicornuate uterus with rudimentary non-functional horn on the left.

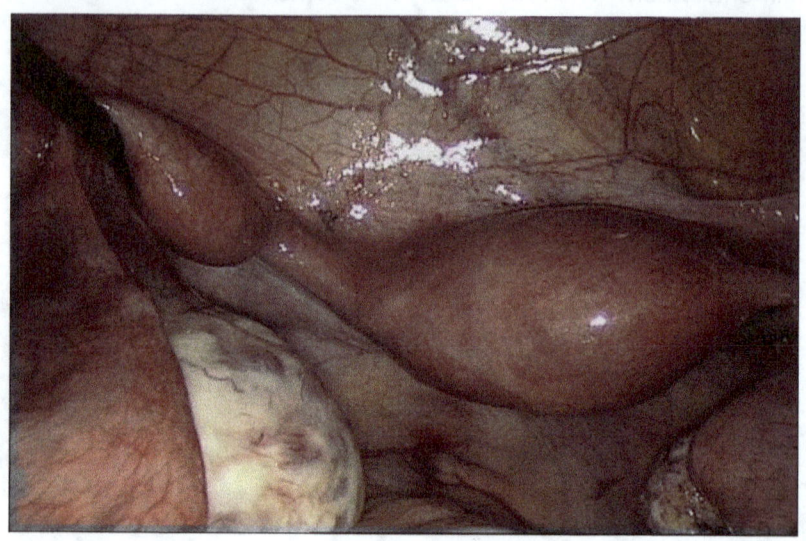

Variant 7c: Unicornuate uterus with normal outline and rudimentary functional endometrial cavity
The endometrial cavity may be connected to the ipsilateral fallopian tube or may even be enclosed.

Variant 7d: Unicornuate uterus with rudimentary non-functional ridge
In cases with an absent or rudimentary horn, a slender rudimentary cord may be detected in the area between the fallopian tube and ovarian and round (broad) ligaments.
Asymmetric uterovaginal variations were found in up to 64% of those with concomitant urinary tract variations (aplasia).
Surgery: laparoscopic removal of the rudimentary horn is recommended in Variants a, b, and d. In rare variant 7c, laparoscopic incision and removal of the endometrial cavity is performed.

Type 8. Septate uterus, incomplete form

Definition – an externally normal uterus with an intermediate uterovaginal septum creating uterine cavities before dividing into an internal cervical ostium, and joining with a single cervical canal; normal vagina.

While the complete intrauterine septum (septate uterus) divides both the uterus and cervical canal, the incomplete intrauterine septum (subseptate uterus begins just from the cervical ostium (Variant 8a) or over (above) the cervical ostium (Variant 8b) and extends to the uterine fundus.

Type 8. Septate uterus, incomplete form (left image).

The intrauterine pregnancy after resection of the uterine septum (right).

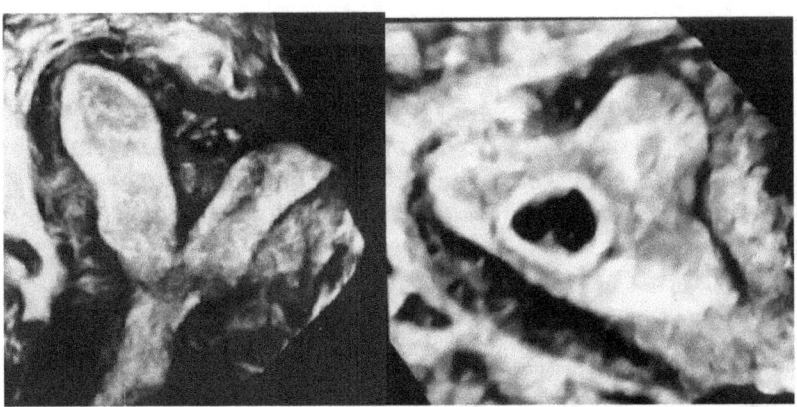

Variant 8a, b: Subseptate uterus (incomplete intrauterine septum)

Incomplete reduction of the intermediate septum during subsequent developmental stages results in a subseptate uterus (or incomplete intrauterine septum). Functional MRI reveals gradual uterine enhancement and a hypersignal. Microcirculation in the septum is reduced by up to 32% in most cases, which explains the high risk of pregnancy loss in 97% of cases. Hysteroresectoscopy identifies poor blood flow in the fibrous septum. Histological morphometry of the septum detects severe reduction and malformation of microcirculatory blood vessels (Makiyan et al., 2016).

Surgery: resection of the incomplete septum in all cases (Variants a and b).

Variant 8c: Residual arcuate septum

The uterovaginal septum is reduced in the last stages of embryogenesis and forms a unicavital uterus. Uterine malformation in these stages results in a persistent residual subseptate arcuate uterus. The external uterus is normally shaped, with an incomplete residual arcuate intrauterine septum.

Surgery: resection of the arcuate residual septum via hysteroresectoscopy in patients with pregnancy losses with elimination of the fibrous tissue with reduced blood perfusion in the uterine fundus.

Variant 8d: Partial (incomplete) uterine and vaginal septum

This atypical form is an extremely rare anatomic variant, where a partial septum persists in the uterine cavity and in the vagina.

Surgery: resection of the both uterine and vaginal septum.

Type 9. Endometrioid uterine cavity (or cystic adenomyosis)

Definition: normal uterus and vagina. Closed, isolated endometrioid uterine cavities have a functional endometrial layer inside.

The endometrioid cavities are usually located where the myometrium crosses the broad uterine ligament or ovarian ligament (which are derivatives of gonadal ridges, like eutopic endometrium). This Type differs from the unicornuate uterus with rudimentary functional endometrial cavity (Variant 7c) in that the Type 9 endometrioid cavity is recognized in the normal uterine cavity and two tubal ostia. The endometrioid uterine cavity (cystic adenomyosis) may be regarded as congenital, because the manifestation begins in young patients from menarche.

Surgery: laparoscopic incision and removal of the endometrial cavity as in variant 7c.

Type 10. Tunnel shaped uterus

Definition: a tunnel shaped or T-shaped uterus characterized by abnormal narrowing of the internal lateral walls of the uterine cavity; normal vagina.
A tunnel shaped or T-shaped uterus is a dysmorphic (dysplastic) uterus that usually co-exists with a "residual arcuate septum" (Variant 8c), these patients classified as having both types (8c and 10), and is characterized by low blood perfusion in the sub-endometrial layer, causing pregnancy loss or infertility.
Surgery: T-shaped uterine cavity enlargement by hysteroresectoscopic section of superficial myometrial layers, performed on bilateral sides and radial (subendometrial) lines.

Type 11. Arcuate uterus

Definition: the external outline of the uterus displays a concave contour into the cavity; normal vagina.

The final stage of uterine development, after reduction of the residual septum, normally results in a genuine arcuate uterus. The uterus is arcuate at birth and becomes normal in shape at puberty under the influence of high estrogen levels. An arcuate uterus in adult females corresponds to genital infantilism and is commonly associated with reproductive failure. These patients require estrogen replacement therapy before pregnancy. Three dimensional (3D) ultrasound or MRI is required for differentiation between genuine arcuate uterus and "residual arcuate septum" (Variant 8c) because management and reproductive outcomes are different. Surgical treatment is not indicated for arcuate uterus.

Type 0. Normal genital anatomy - No structural variations

Definition: normally shaped unicavital uterus and vagina.

Discussion

While some anatomical variations are immediately obvious on external examination of the newborn, many internal variations are not diagnosed until much later. Internal examination of the genital morphology of newborns and young adolescents should be considered in cases where anatomical variations are suspected. Currently, three dimensional (3D) ultrasound examination (intra-abdominal or transrectal) is most important for evaluation of internal organ anatomy. Vaginoscopic inspection with a small tube and camera may be useful for detecting variations in adolescent females who present with vaginal aplasia and menstrual outflow obstruction. Functional (DCE) MRI in patients with symmetric variations enables evaluation of areas with reduced blood perfusion and is important for surgical treatment and embryo transfer in an IVF program. Reproductive surgery in patients with uterine variations depends on blood perfusion parameters to create a normally shaped uterine cavity and eliminate areas with reduced blood perfusion, thereby preventing reproductive losses.

An international database of congenital diseases may be the best platform for unifying practice expertise from global clinicians, enabling collection of statistical data and a consensus statement for management of genital organ variations (anomalies). Each patient with a congenital anomaly would be assigned an individual identifier code (digital ID) for anonymous database registration and statistical evaluation. New data for under-reported congenital variations (anomalies), which may be diagnosed later in life, will aid in increasing our understanding of these conditions and their optimal treatment. An upgraded statistical system based on this new information may lead to universal guidance for screening, surgical treatment, and rehabilitation in females with congenital variations of the reproductive organs.

This new classification of uterovaginal variations according to anatomic types and embryonic developmental stages provides a much more robust system for identifying and managing these cases. Appropriate management and optimal surgical treatment of female genital variations will improve reproductive health and outcomes for a new generation.

Table II-1. New Classification and Management for Uterovaginal Anatomic Variants

Type	Uterovaginal variants	Management and Surgery
1a	Uterine and vaginal aplasia with non-functional rudiments	Laparoscopy, removal of the uterine rudiments, creation of neovagina
1b	Uterine and vaginal aplasia with functional rudiments	Laparoscopy, removal of the uterine rudiments, creation of neovagina
2a	Cervicovaginal agenesis, rudimental uterus	Laparoscopy, cervicovaginal stentation
2b	Cervicovaginal aplasia, functional uterus	Laparoscopy, cervicovaginal stentation or anastomosis
3a	Partial vaginal aplasia	Vaginoplasty, laparoscopy recommended
3b	Hymen imperforatum	Hymenoplasty
4a	Double uterus and vagina, symmetric	Resection of the vaginal septum, functional MRI for estimation of the hemiuteri with better blood perfusion in IVF program
4b	Double uterus and vagina asymmetric, with partial aplasia of hemivagina	Laparoscopy for evacuation of retrograde menstrual flow, resection of the common vaginal septum
5a	Completely septate uterus and cervical canal	Hysteroresectoscopy, resection of vaginal, cervical and uterine septum
5b	Completely septate uterus, double cervix	Hysteroresectoscopy, resection of intrauterine and vaginal septum, double cervix preserved
6	Bicornuate uterus (**6a**, complete and **6b**, incomplete form)	3-D ultrasound or MRI to verify anatomy
7a	Unicornuate uterus with rudimentary horn with functional endometrial cavity	Laparoscopy, removal of the rudimental horns
7b	Unicornuate uterus with rudimentary non-functional horn	Laparoscopy, removal of the rudimental horns
7c	Unicornuate uterus with normal outline and rudimentary functional endometrial cavity	Laparoscopy, incision of endometrial cavity
7d	Unicornuate uterus with rudimentary non-functional ridge	Laparoscopy, removal of the rudimental ridge
8a, b	Subseptate uterus (incomplete intrauterine septum)	Hysteroresectoscopy, resection of intrauterine septum
8c	Arcuate residual septum	Hysteroresectoscopy, resection of residual septum
8d	Partial uterine/vaginal septum	Resection of septum
9	Endometrioid uterine cavity (cystic adenomyosis)	Laparoscopy, incision of endometrial cavity
10	Tunnel or T-shaped uterus	Hysteroresectoscopic enlargement of uterine cavity
11	Arcuate uterus, genital infantilism (uterine hypoplasia)	Estrogen replacement treatment

Figure II-1. Anatomic Classification of Uterovaginal Variations. Schematic patterns of anomalous types.

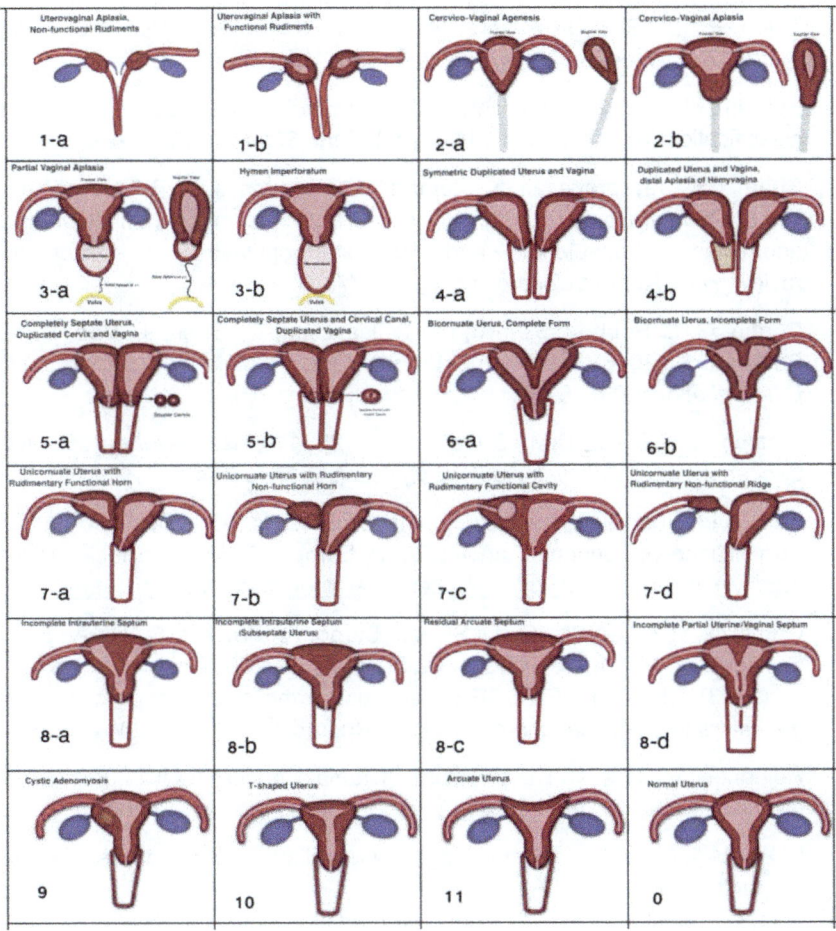

References

Acién, P., & Acién, M. (2016a). The presentation and management of complex female genital malformations. *Hum Reprod Update*. 22(1), 48–69.

Acién, P. (2016b). On a New Neovaginal Prosthesis of PLA (Polylactic Acid). *Am J Pharmacol Pharmacother*. 3(2), 16-19.

Buttram, V.C., & Gibbons, W.E. (1979). Mullerian anomalies: a proposed classification (an analysis of 144 cases). *Fertil Steril*. 32(1), 40–46.

Chan, Y.Y., Jayaprakasan, K., Zamora, J., Thornton, J.G., Raine-Fenning, N., & Coomarasamy, A. (2011). The prevalence of congenital uterine anomalies in unselected and high-risk populations: a systematic review. *Hum Reprod Update*. 17(6), 761-771.

Cunha, G.R., Robboy, S.J., Kurita, T., Isaacson, D., Shen, J., Cao, M., & Baskin, L.S. (2018). Development of the human female reproductive tract. *Differentiation*. 103, 46–65.

Dietrich, J.E., Millar, D.M., & Quint, E.H. (2014). Obstructive reproductive tract anomalies. *J Pediatr Adolesc Gynecol*. 27(6), 396-402.

European Surveillance of Congenital Anomalies (EUROCAT). (2017). Surveillance of congenital anomalies in Europe. Prevalence table. URL: http://www.eurocat-network.eu/accessprevalencedata/prevalencetables.

Grimbizis, G.F., Gordts, S., Di Spiezio Sardo, A., Brucker, S., De Angelis, C., Gergolet, M., Li, T.C., Tanos, V., Brölmann, H., Gianaroli, L., & Campo, R. (2013). The ESHRE/ESGE consensus on the classification of female genital tract congenital anomalies. Hum Reprod. 28(8), 2032-2044.

Heinonen, P.K. (2016). Distribution of female genital tract anomalies in two classifications. *Eur J Obstet Gynecol Reprod Biol*. 206, 141-146.

Hill, M.A. (2020). Embryology Australian abnormalities 81-92 urogenital.jpg. URL: https://embryology.med.unsw.edu.au/embryology/index.php/File:Australian_abnormalities_81-92_urogenital.jpg.

Isaacson, D., Shen, J., Overland, M., Li, Y., Sinclair, A., Cao, M., McCreedy, D., Calvert, M., McDevitt, T., Cunha, G.R., & Baskin, L. (2018). Three-dimensional imaging of the developing human fetal urogenital-genital tract: Indifferent stage to male and female differentiation. *Differentiation.* 103, 14-23. doi: 10.1016/j.diff.2018.09.003.

Makiyan, Z.N., Adamyan, L.V., Bychenko, V.G., Miroshnikova, N.A., & Kozlova, A.V. (2016). Functional magnetic resonance imaging for the determination of blood flow in symmetric uterine anomalies. *Obstet Gynecol Moscow.* 10, 73-79.

Makiyan, Z. (2016a). Studies of gonadal sex differentiation. *Organogenesis.* 12(1), 42-51.

Makiyan, Z. (2016b). Systematization of ambiguous genitalia. *Organogenesis.* 12(4), 169-182.

Matthews, T.J., MacDorman, M.F., & Thoma, M.E. (2015). Infant mortality statistics from the 2013 period linked birth/infant death data set. *Natl Vital Stat Rep.* 64(9), 1-30.

Monlleó. I.L., Zanotti, S.V., de Araújo, B.P.B., Júnior, E.F.C., Pereira, P.D., de Barros, P.M., Araújo, M.D.P., de Mendonça, A.T.V., Santos, C.R., dos Santos, Y.R. & de Paula Michelatto, D. (2012). Prevalence of genital abnormalities in neonates. *J Pediatr (Rio J).* 88(6), 489-495.

Paradisi, R., Barzanti, R., & Fabbri, R. (2014). The techniques and outcomes of hysteroscopic metroplasty. *Curr Opin Obstet Gynecol.* 26(4), 295-301.

Prior, M., Richardson, A., Asif, S., Polanski, L., Parris-Larkin, M., Chandler, J., Fogg, L., Jassal, P., Thornton, J.G., & Raine-Fenning, N.J. (2018). Outcome of assisted reproduction in women with congenital uterine anomalies: a prospective observational study. *Ultrasound Obstet Gynecol.* 51(1), 110-117.

Rezaei, Z., Omidvar, A., Niroumanesh, S., & Omidvar, A. (2015). Cervicovaginal anastomosis by Gore-Tex in Mullerian agenesis. *Arch Gynecol Obstet.* 291(2), 467-472.

World Health Organisation (WHO). (2018). International Classification of Diseases for Mortality and Morbidity Statistics (ICD-11). 2018 version. URL: http://id.who.int/icd/entity/2013857037

III. NEW THEORY OF UTEROVAGINAL EMBRYOGENESIS

Introduction

The explanation of the uterine and vaginal embryogenesis in humans still poses many controversies, because it is difficult to assess early stages of an embryo.

Professor Johannes Peter Muller was the furst comparative anatomist, who investigated by simple light microscopy early human embryonic stages and described developmental theory in 1830.

According to the original Mullerian theory (Fig. III-1): "Gonads appear as a pair of longitudinal ridges on the dorsolateral sides. Immediately below of the gonadal ridges the mesonephral ducts (Wollfian) grow caudally (on the medial part).

The paramesonephral (so called Müllerian ducts) develop autonomously and parallel to the paramedial parts of the mesonephral.

The mesonephral ducts regress in female embryos; paramesonephral ducts form the Fallopian tubes, uterus and vagina".

According to Mullerian (1830) theory, initially two pairs of genital ducts, mesonephral (Wolffian) and paramesonephral (Mullerian), form in both sexes.

In female embryo, the two paramesonephral (Mullerian) ducts are conjoined in the midline in the caudo-cranial direction. There are separated by an intermediate septum. The intermediate uterovaginal septum decreases and fuses into a single canal, forming the unicavital (normal) uterus and vagina. The Fallopian tubes, uterus and vagina develop from pairs of paramesonephral (Mullerian) ducts. The vestibulum vaginae completely derive from

63

the sinus urogenitalis. Although the mesonephros and mesonephral ducts form rete testis and seminiferous ducts in males, they reduce in females. [1, 2]

Fig. III-1. Müller JP. Bildungsgeschichte der Genitalien. Düsseldorf: Arnz, 1830; 185-187.

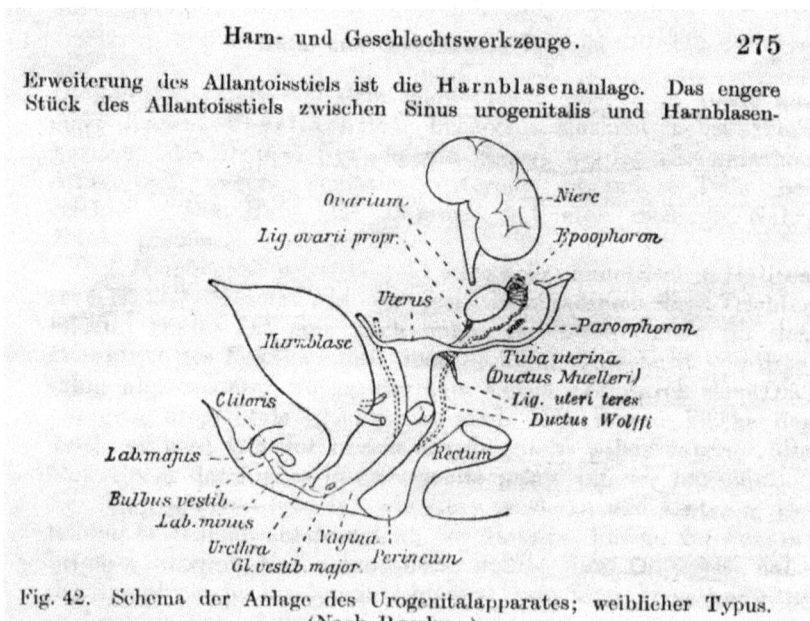

The literature review revealed many disagreements in Mullerian theory, inciting some authors to propose new embryological hypotheses.

In most textbooks, the contemporary theories of uterovaginal development show some differences, considering the dual origin of vagina. The Fallopian tubes, uterus and proximal 1/3 of the vagina derive from the paramesonephral ducts. The vestibulum vaginae and distal 2/3 of the vagina derive from the urogenital sinus. [3-9]

Several authors had researched the origin of the vagina, they considered this issue has been insufficiently studied.

Clinical evidences

Developmental uterovaginal anomalies (named after Mullerian) result from the influence of teratogenous lesions during critical periods of morphogenesis, each variant of them corresponds to persistent normal embryonic development stages.

The early stage of embryonal development corresponds to uterovaginal aplasia (Fig. III-2).

Figure III-2. The right non-functional uterine rudiment in patient with uterovaginal aplasia.

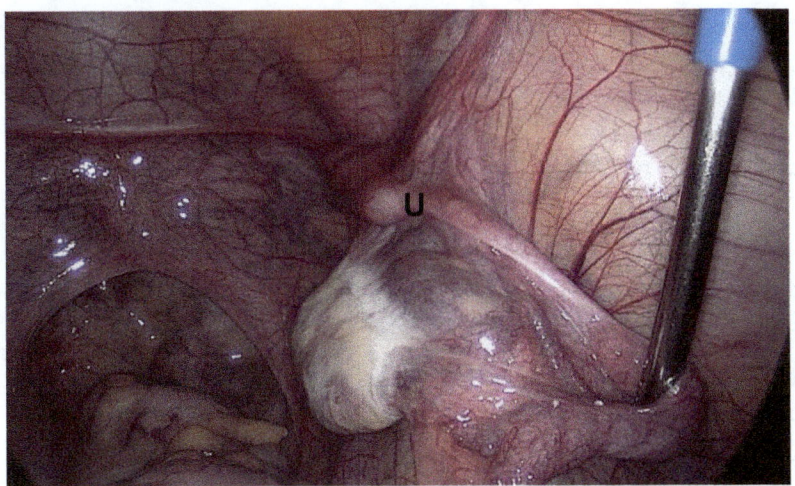

O – ovary, F – Fallopian tube, LO – ligamentum ovaricum proprium, LT – ligamentum teres uteri, U – uterine rudiment

During laparoscopy, all patients with uterovaginal aplasia (MRKH syndrome) had rudimentary uterine horns. The non-functional rudiments had 73% patients, approximately 20x12x15 mm in size (derivatives of Mullerian ducts) and normally shaped Fallopian tubes and ovaries. Both rudimentary horns were detected in the crossing area between the Fallopian tubes, with round ligaments and ovarian ligaments.

The functional uterine rudiments with endometrial cavities had 17% patients, which removed laparoscopically.

Fusion defects of Mullerian ducts result in symmetric malformations: duplicate uterus and vagina, bicornuate uterus, and septate uterus. [1, 2, 6]

The clinical cases of completely duplicate uterus and vagina possibly arose during the developing stages of paired Mullerian ducts before their fusion.

These cases of fully duplicate vagina triggered controversy over contemporary views that describe the origin of the proximal 1/3 part of the vagina from paramesonephral (Mullerian) ducts and the distal 2/3 from the sinus urogenitalis. The urogenital sinus, as a part of the cloaca, is an unpaired structure.

Later, the pair of Mullerian ducts fuses together and the intermediate uterovaginal septum separates into two uterine cavities and cervical canals. Persistence of this stage corresponds to a completely septate uterus.

Uterine malformation during subsequent stages results in a subseptate uterus.

The uterovaginal septum reduces and finally forms the unicavital normal uterus.

The last stage of uterine development, after the reduction of the intermediate septum, is an arcuate uterus. The normally shaped uterus becomes under the influence of high estrogen levels.

Distal aplasia of 1/3 or 2/3 of the vagina with obstruction of menstrual outflow are due to vaginal outgrowth defects of the cloaca.

Complete cervico-vaginal aplasia with functional uterus suppose the controversy of "unidirectional" caudo-cranial theory of Mullerian ducts fusion.

Hymen imperforatum – is the last stage of vaginal connection onto the cloaca. Normally, the hymenal septum between vagina and vestibulum vaginae perforates due to physiological apoptosis (O'Rahilly, 1977). [5]

The vestibulum vaginae had normal anatomy in all of the patients with uterovaginal aplasia (MRKH syndrome), partial or complete vaginal aplasia, or fully duplicated vagina. This demonstrated that the vestibulum vaginae derive from the sinus urogenitalis. [1, 2]

According to embryological data, the ureters and permanent kidneys develop from ureteric buds as outgrowths of the distal part of mesonephral ducts close to the entrance of the cloaca. [8]

A high (12%) incidence of renal abnormalities was found in patients with uterine malformations.

Clinical analysis estimates that unicornuate uterus is associated with ipsilateral renal aplasia in 64% of cases, whereas duplicated uterus and vagina, with partial aplasia of the hemyvagina, is associated with ipsilateral renal aplasia in all (100%) cases.

Because all cases of unilateral renal agenesis are associated with ipsilateral blind vagina, it has been hypothesized that the vagina derives from themesonephral (not the paramesonephral) ducts.

Experimental evidences

We found some very important evidences in the literature and in contemporary embryological investigations confirming the new proposed theory about uterovaginal embryogenesis.

Sanchez-Ferrer M. et al. (2006) immunohystochemically investigated the "experimental contributions to the study of the embryology of the vagina" in rats and found that the human vagina derives from the mesonephral ducts. [21]

In accordance with contemporary embryology, the male prostatic utricle is a rudimentary analog of the female uterus. The prostatic utricle is believed to be a remnant of the fused caudal ends of the paramesonephral ducts. [3, 6, 7]

Shapiro E et al (2004) used immunohystochemical probes and provided strong evidence that "the prostatic utricle is not a Mullerian duct remnant" but of a urogenital sinus origin. [25]

Recent embryological investigations with electronic microscopy have revealed some nuances: the mesonephral ducts are located on the external part of the mesonephros and at the paramedial sides of the gonadal ridges.

The very important histological images represented at the website of the embryological unit at University of New South Wales, Sydney, Australia (Fig. III-3) [Dr. Mark Hill, Embryology, 2022. https://embryology.med.unsw.edu.au/embryology/index.php/Main_Page]

Figure III-3. Histological image of pig embryo on Carnegie stage 13 (equal to the day 42 human embryo).
https://embryology.med.unsw.edu.au/embryology/index.php/File:Stage_13_image_093.jpg

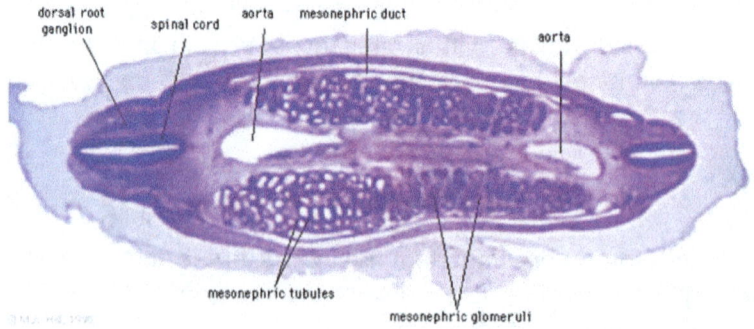

At the histological images of the human female embryo on Carnegie stage 22 (which is approximately equal to week 8 of development), the mesonephral ducts are also located on the paramedial sides (Fig. III-4).

Figure III-4. Histological images of human female embryo on Carnegie stage 22.
https://embryology.med.unsw.edu.au/embryology/index.php/File:Stage_22_image_214.jpg

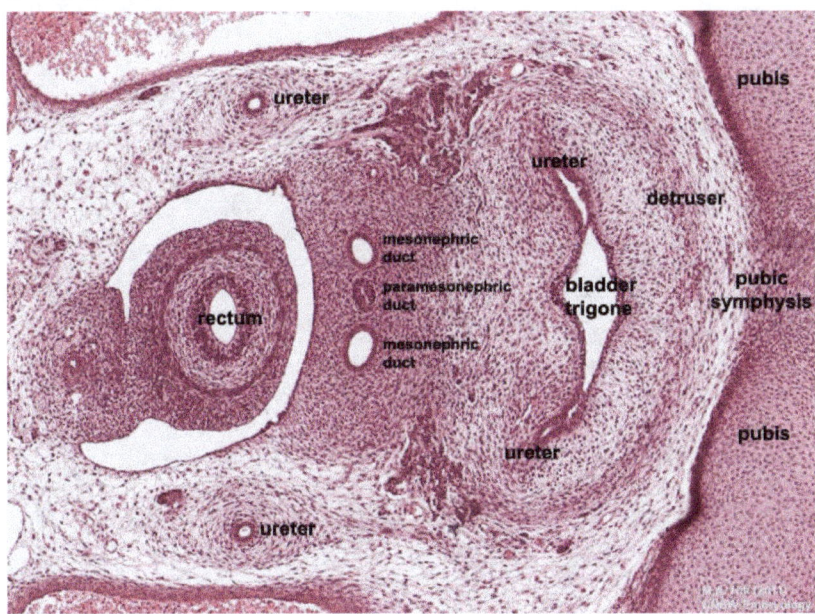

The so-called paramesonephric ducts at this image are located at medial sides, and probably correspond to gonadal ridges. [6]

Hurst C et al (2002), investigated in utero exposure to 2,3,7,8-tetrachlorodibenzo-p-dioxin (TCDD) during the critical periods of female rats organogenesis. In support of our new theory, there is evidence of uterine development in the area of intersection between mesonephral ducts with gonadal ridges and fusion of both uterine folds. Figure III-4 shows that there are two Mullerian ducts fusing with Wolffian ducts separately on the left and right sides in the early stage of gestation (GD 18 and 19) (Fig. III-5 A, C). Then, on GD 21, both duct pairs fused and conjoined with one another on their medial parts (Fig. III-5 A, C). [26]

Fig. III-5. Hurst CH, Abbott B, Schmid JE, Birnbaum LS. Feulgen staining of female rat reproductive tracts after GD 15 administration of 1.0 µg TCDD/kg showing width of interductal mesenchyme.

[Toxicol Sci, Volume 65, Issue 1, January 2002, Pages 87–98, https://doi.org/10.1093/toxsci/65.1.87]

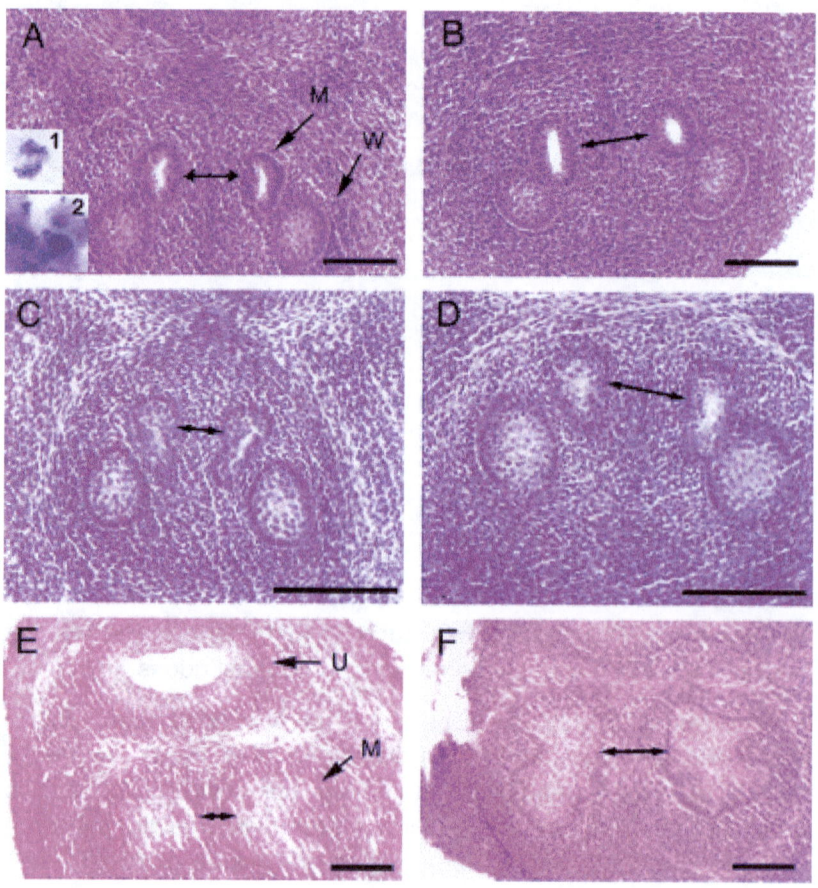

In the IX-th edition of Langman's Medical Embryology (Sadler, 2000; page 324, Fig. 14.3 C), there is an electron micrograph of a mouse female embryo (Fig. III-6) showing the genital ridges (white arrows) growing immediately below of the gonads. Mesonephos (black arrowheads) and their ureters - mesonephral ducts are located on the paramedial sides of the mesonephros. [3]

Accepting, that the early stages of embryonal development correspond to uterovaginal aplasia (Fig. III-2), we could compare this electron micrograph (Fig. III-6) with anatomy of the uterine rudiments in patient with uterovaginal aplasia. It seems that the uterine folds (U) (red doted rings) are situated in crossing area between mesonephral ducts with gonadal ridges.

Hashimoto (2003) in a study of human embryos development by electron microscopy on Carnegie stages 18-23, detected the active cell-to-cell communications between the Mullerian and Wolffian cells. [27]

Figure III-6. The electron micrograph of a mouse female embryo on undifferentiated stage. In the IX-th edition of Langman's Medical Embryology. G – gonads. The uterine folds are located in the area of intersection between mesonephral ducts with gonadal ridges (red rings)

[Courtesy of Dr. K.K. Sulik. Department of Cell and Developmental Biology, University of North Carolina]

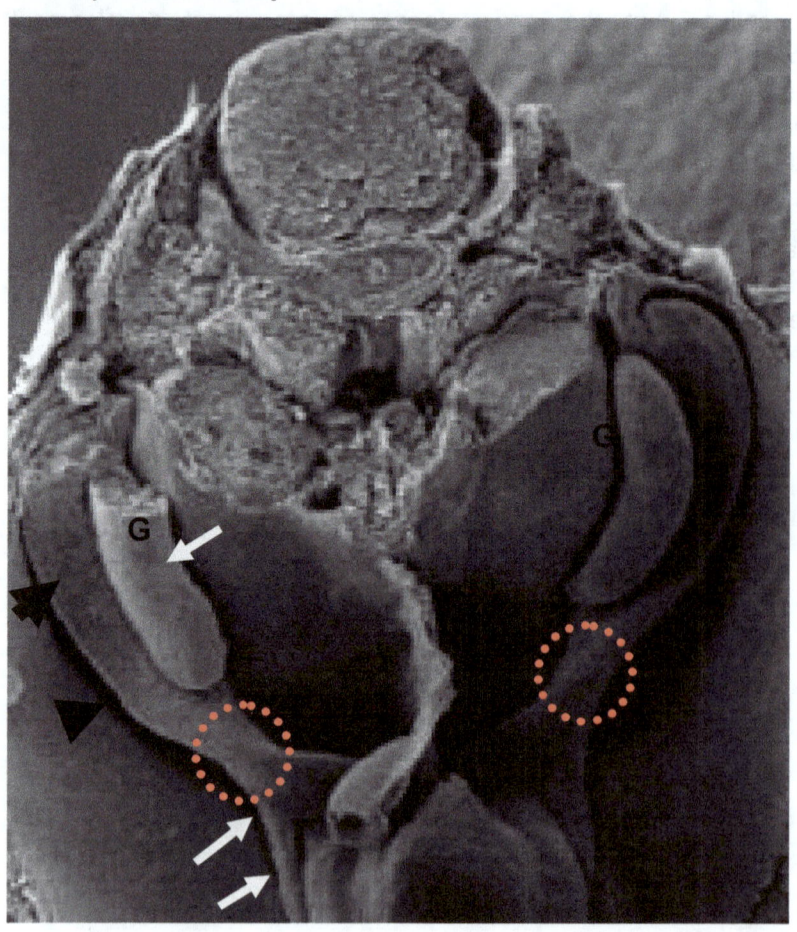

Discussion

The new theory which is proposed in this chapter may be explain the process of normal uterovaginal embryogenesis and the abnormal development of the presented clinical cases.

The key differences between existing and the proposed new hypothesis are follows (Table III-1):

1. in original Mullerian theory the mesonephral ducts regress in female embryos (Fig. III-1, Fig. III-7);

paramesonephral ducts form the Fallopian tubes, uterus and vagina;

2. in new theory (Fig. III-8) the mesonephral ducts in female embryos form Fallopian tubes, and vagina; the uterus derive in crossing area between mesonephral ducts with gonadal ridges.

Hence, the paramesonephral ducts do not exist.

Although the origin of the Mullerian duct is unknown, according to most textbooks, the Mullerian ducts develop autonomously as an invagination of the coelomic epithelium.
The detailed study with electronic microscopy revealed that the paramedial ducts (so called Mullerian) actually – the mesonephral ducts.

Thus the Mullerian ducts have mesonephric origin (not from coelomic epitelium).

Accordingly of the New theory of uterovaginal embryogenesis:
The medial located ducts (Wollfian) – correspond with Gonadal ridges. The paramedial (Mullerian) ducts – in fact appear as the mesonephral ducts.
The paramesonephral ducts are absent.

The hypothetic possibility that the ovary and endometrium derive from the gonadal ridges could be the key to understanding the enigmatic aetiologies of extra-genital and ovarian endometriosis (Chapter IV).

Table III-1.

Derivative organs	Original Mullerian theory	Contemporary view	Theory by Makiyan
Gonads	gonadal ridge	gonadal ridge	gonadal ridge
Ligamentum ovaricum			gonadal ridge derivatives
Ligamentum teres uteri	paramesonephral ducts		gonadal ridge derivatives
Fallopian tubes	paramesonephral ducts	paramesonephral ducts	mesonephral ducts
Uterus	paramesonephral ducts	paramesonephral ducts	fusion of the gonadal ridges with mesonephral ducts
Vagina	paramesonephral ducts	proximal 1/3 from paramesonephral ducts, distal 2/3 – from urogenital sinus	mesonephral ducts
Vestibulum vaginae	sinus urogenitalis	distal part of sinus urogenitalis	sinus urogenitalis

Fig. III-7. Mullerian Theory: the paramesonephral ducts (red color) form uterus vagina; the mesonephral ducts are reduced (grey color).

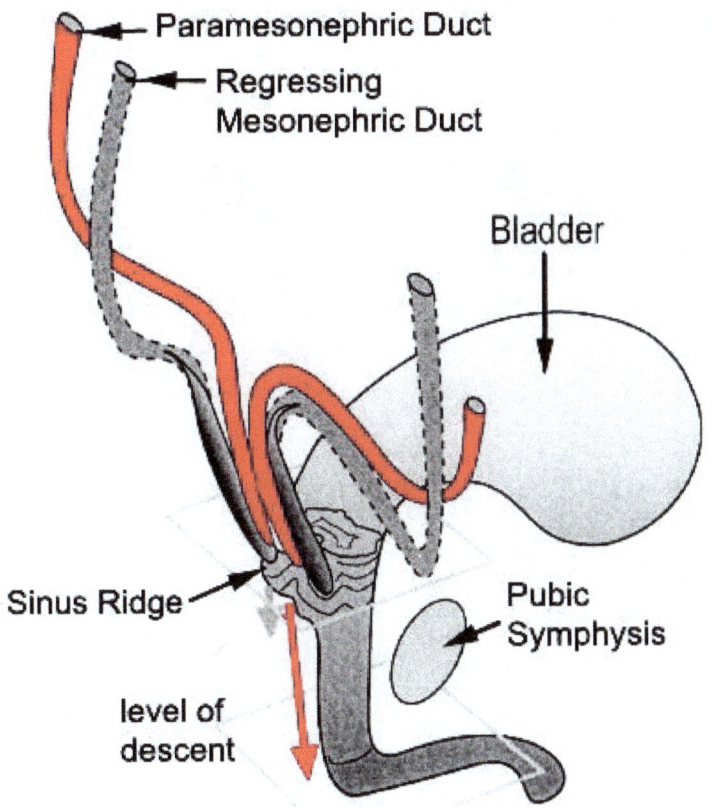

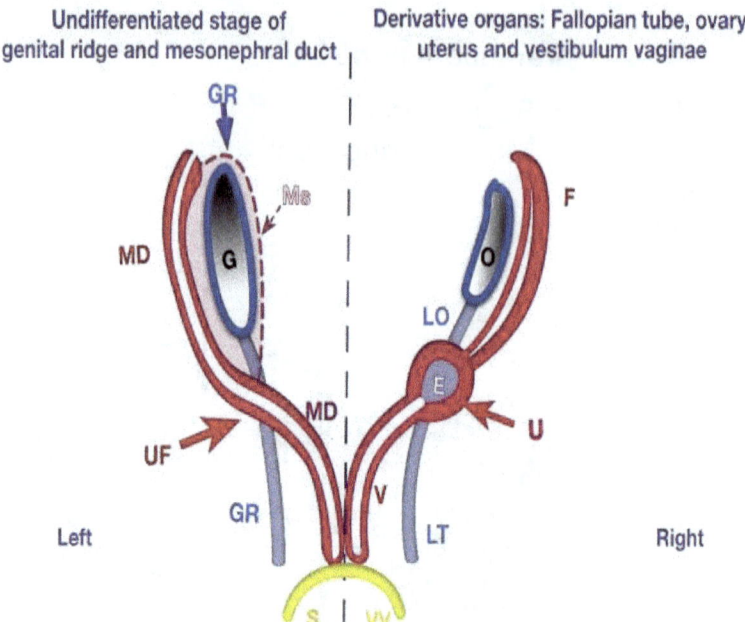

Fig. III-8. Makiyan Z. New theory of uterovaginal embryogenesis.

References

1. Müller JP. Bildungsgeschichte der Genitalien. Düsseldorf: Arnz, 1830; 185-187.

2. Muller JP. Anatomie des Menschen. Berlin: Miller, 1931; 272-275.

3. Sadler TW. "Langman's Medical Embryology". IX-th edn, Baltimore: Lippincott Williams&Wilkins, 2000; 324, Fig. 14.3-C.

   https://archive.org/stream/LangmansMedicalEmbryology#page/n342/mode/1up

4. O'Rahilly R, Müller F. Embryologie und Teratologie des Menschen. Huber Verlag 1999; 107-109.

5. O'Rahilly R. The development of the vagina in the human. In: RJ Blandau& D Bergsmall (eds) Morphogenesis and Malformation of the Genital System. Birth Defects. New York: Alan Liss 1977; 123–136.

6. Hill M.A. (2014) Embryology BGD Lecture - Sexual Differentiation. Retrieved October 16, 2014. URL: http://php.med.unsw.edu.au/embryology/index.php?title=BGD_Lecture_Sexual_Differentiation

7. Jost AA. The new look at the mechanism controlling sex differentiation in mammals. Johns Hopkins Medical Journal 1972; 130: 28-36.

8. Sadler TW. "Langman's Medical Embryology". XII-th edn, Baltimore: Lippincott Williams&Wilkins, 2012; 232-259.

9. Acién P. Embryological observations on the female genital tract. Hum Reprod 1992;7:437–445.

10. Acién P, Susarte F, Romero J, et al. Complex genital malformation: ectopic ureter ending in a supposed mesonephric duct in a woman with renal agenesis and ipsilateral blind hemivagina. Eur J Obstet Gynecol Reprod Biol 2004; Nov 10;117(1):105-8.

11. Acien P, Arminana E, Garcia-Ontiveros E. Unilateral renal agenesis associated with ipsilateral blind vagina. Arch Gynecol 1987;240:1—8.

12. Acien P, Acien M, Sanchez-Ferrer M. Complex malformations of the female genital tract. New types and revision of classification. Hum Reprod 2004 Nov 10;117(1):105-8. doi: 10.1093/humrep/deh423

13. Acién P, Acién M. Unilateral renal agenesis and female genital tract pathologies. Acta Obstet Gynecol Scand. 2010 Nov;89(11):1424-31. doi: 10.3109/00016349.2010.512067.

14. Sanchez-Ferrer M, Acien M, Sanchez Del Campo, Mayol-Belda M, Acién P. Experimental contributions to the study of the embryology of the vagina. Hum Reprod. Embryol 2006;21:6. doi: 10.1093/humrep/del031

15. Fritsch H, Richter E, Adam N. Molecular characteristics and alterations during early development of the human vagina. Journal of Anatomy. Vol. 220, Issue 4, pp. 363–371, April 2012. doi: 10.1111/j.1469-7580.2011.01472.x

16. The American Fertility Society classification of adnexal adhesions, distal tubal occlusion, tubal occlusion secondary to tubal ligation, tubal pregnancies, Mullerian anomalies and intrauterine adhesions. Fertil Steril 1988; Jun;49(6):944-55.

17. Grimbizis GF, Gordts S, Di Spiezio Sardo A, et al. T he ESHRE/ESGE consensus on the classification of female genital tract congenital anomalies. Hum Reprod 2013 Aug;28(8):2032-44. doi: 10.1093/humrep/det098.

18. Musset R, Mu¨ller P, Netter A. et al. Etat du haut appareil urinaire chez les porteuses de malformations uterines: etude de 133 observations. Presse Med 1967;75:1331–1336.

19. Fatum M, Rojansky N, Shushan A. Septate uterus with cervical duplication: rethinking the development of Mullerian anomalies. Gynecol Obstet Invest 2003;55:3:186-188. doi:10.1159/000071535

20. Martínez-Frías ML, Frías JL, Opitz JM. Errors of morphogenesis and developmental field theory. Am J Med Genet 1998, 76: 291-296. doi: 10.1002/(SICI)1096-8628(19980401)76:4<291::AID-AJMG3>3.0.CO;2-T

21. Giraldo JL, Habana A, Duleba AJ, Dokras A. Septate uterus associated with cervical duplication and vaginal septum. J Am Assoc Gynecol Laparosc 2000 May;7(2):277-9.

22. Shapiro E, Huang H, McFadden D, et al. The prostatic utricle is not a Mullerian duct remnant: immunonistochemical evidence for a distinct urogenital sinus origin. J Urol. 2004; 172: 1753-1756. http://dx.doi.org/10.1097/01.ju.0000140267.46772.7d

23. Hurst CH, Abbott B, Schmid JE, Birnbaum LS. Feulgen staining of female rat reproductive tracts after GD 15 administration of 1.0 μg TCDD/kg showing width of interductal mesenchyme. Toxicol Sci. Published online: Jan 2002. doi: 10.1093/toxsci/65.1.87. Available from URL: http://toxsci.oxfordjournals.org/content/65/1/87/F6.expansion.html

24. Grimbizis GF, Campo R; on Behalf of the SC of the CONUTA ESHRE/ESGE Working Group, Gordts G, Brucker S, Gergolet M, Tanos V, Li T-C, De Angelis C, Di Spiezio Sardo A. Clinical approach for the classification of congenital uterine malformations. Gynecol Surg 2012;9:119–129.

25. Signorile PG, Baldi A. 2010a. Endometriosis: New concepts in the pathogenesis. Int J Biochem Cell Biol 42: 778-780.

26. Knapp VJ. 1999. How old is endometriosis? Late 17th and 18th century European descriptions of the disease. Fertil Steril 72: 10-14.

IV. ENDOMETRIUM ORIGINATING FROM PRIMORDIAL GERM CELLS

Introduction

The primary question is determining the origin of eutopic (normally cited) endometrium.

The origin of the normaly cited endometrium is currently unknown.

The second question to understanding the etiology of endometrial ectopia (endometriosis) is determining the origin of eutopic (normally cited) endometrium.

Endometriosis is defined as the presence of ectopic endometrial glands and stroma outside of the uterine cavity. [1, 2]

Multiple hypotheses have been postulated to explain the etiology of endometriosis to understand various clinical evidences. The etiology of endometriosis is still unclear.

External endometrial lesions are frequently found in the pelvic peritoneum (extra-genital endometriosis) and ovaries (ovarian cyst or superficial heterotopies). Most often, external endometriosis is located on the peritoneal surface of the recto-vaginal space: at the retrocervical area, on the uterosacral ligaments and in the recto-sigmoid region of the colon. Endometrial lesions can also be found at scars of the abdominal wall; on the bladder and ureters, and on the bowels and appendix. Rarely, endometriosis is recognized in other extra abdominal organs, such as the brain and oculus. [1, 2]

Internal endometriosis (adenomyosis) is characterized by the presence of heterotopic endometrial glands and stroma in the uterine intramural muscular layer (deep in the myometrium) and is surrounded by reactive fibrosis of the myocytes. [1-3]

Endometriosis is a proliferative estrogen dependent disorder; symptoms may begin in adolescence. The prevalence of endometriosis in the female population is estimated to be 6 to 10%, and the frequency increases to 24–35% in females with pain and up to 50–60% in women with infertility. [1-3]

The most often symptoms are refers to endometriosis: chronic pelvic pain, algodysmenorrhea, dyspareunia and primary infertility. Congenital uterovaginal anomalies defined as rare conditions that represent in 4–7% females, [1-4] however the concomitant endometriosis revealed in 46% of those cases.

The extra-genital endometriosis was the major concomitant pathology revealed in 46% patients with uterovaginal anomalies with obstruction of menstrual outflow (partial or complete vaginal aplasia, functional uterine horn) and in non-obstructive symmetric malformations (uterus duplex, septate uterus).

The prevalence of the extra-genital endometriosis in female population is 6–10%; the frequency increases to 35–60% in women with pain, infertility or uterovaginal malformations. For a review see refs. [28–30]

Some authors have reported endometriosis in patients with complete utero-vaginal aplasia. [31, 32]

Signorile et al. investigated the autopsies of (101) human female fetuses at different gestational ages and found ectopic endometrium in 9% of cases.5,6 The authors suggested that endometriosis developed during organogenesis by dislocation (ectopia) of primitive endometrial tissue outside of the uterine cavity. [7]

Jean Bouquet de Jolinière et al. researched the reproductive organs from 7 female fetuses at autopsy between 18 and 36 weeks of gestation. Serial sections revealed numerous ectopic endometrial glands and embryonic duct remnants inside the myometrium, uterine broad and ovarian ligaments and under the fallopian tube serosa in 2 fetuses with low levels of expression of estrogen receptor-α (ER-a) and progesterone receptors (PR). Authors have supported the theory that some subtypes of endometrioid lesions may be related to anomalies occurring during embryogenesis. [8]

Male endometriosis of the prostate and male "uterus-like mass" are 2 unusual manifestations of endometriosis. González RS et al. [10] reported a case of male uterus-like mass (endomyometriosis) in the right inguinal area at the site of a prior hernia repair. The lesion was tubular in shape, with a thick muscular wall and a central blood-filled lumen. Microscopically, the tissue showed layers of concentric smooth muscle, with endometrial glands and stroma lining the lumen. [9, 10]

How explain the presence of endometriosis: in female fetuses, in females with complete utero-vaginal aplasia without functional endometrial cavity and even in males or DSD (disorders of sex development) patients with 46,XY karyotype?

The goal of this article is to understanding the etiology of endometriosis and presence of endometrioid lesions in unusual cases.

Endometriosis theories

Multiple hypotheses (Table IV-1) have been postulated to explain the etiology of endometriosis to understand various clinical evidences in females.

The Implantation theory of endometriosis is the most widely accepted. Sampson proposes that reflux or retrograde menstruation allowing outflow of endometrial tissue through the Fallopian tubes into the abdominal cavity is followed by implantation of endometrial glands and stroma at extra-uterine sites. [11]

The coelomic metaplasia theory suggests metaplastic processes of the peritoneal mesothelium in endometriosis. [12]

The metaplasia theory supports the transformation of the germinal epithelium into ovarian endometriosis. [13]

Circulating stem cells are proposed to be involved in the transformation of pluripotent haematopoietic stem cells in endometrial cells in the peritoneal cavity. [14, 15]

Knapp postulated that endometriosis is caused by small defects of embryogenesis. Mullerian duct maldevelopment during embryogenesis could cause the spread of endometriotic cells across the posterior pelvic floor and the persistence of embryonic cell rests. [4]

Lymphatic and vascular dissemination theories have been proposed to explain the presence of endometrial lesions in lymphatic vessels and the spread to lymph nodes and rare sites. [16]

Immune dysfunction and deficiency impair the survival of endometrial cells and lesion establishment, and high reoccurrence rates occur following treatment. Additionally, lymph-angiogenesis in endometriotic lesions may contribute to lesion growth and persistence of endometrial cells in the draining lymph nodes. [17, 18]

Adenomyosis may originate from the invagination of the basalis of the endometrium into the myometrium. As a second theory, this basalis invagination proceeds along the intra-myometrial lymphatic system. A third theory suggests that a metaplastic process initiating from ectopic intramyometrial endometrial tissue is produced de novo. [3,18-20]

Many theories have been proposed regarding the etiology of both endomyometriosis and endometriosis in males, including remnant areas of Müllerian tissue and metaplasia. [3, 9, 10, 13, 15]

Various theories have also been combined to understand the unusual types of endometriosis. Although its underlying cause is uncertain, it is likely to be multifactorial and include genetic factors with possible epigenetic influences, hormonal induction and apoptosis suppression. [18-20]

Table IV-1. Various theories of endometriosis aetiology.

Theory	Mechanism
Implantation theory	Retrograde menstruation allowing implantation of endometrial glands in pelvic peritoneum
Coelomic metaplasia	Transformation of peritoneal mesothelium or other cell types into endometrial tissue
Hormonal induction	Oestrogen-driven proliferation of endometrial lesions or metaplasia by hormonal stimulation
Inflammation and oxidative stress	Recruitment of immune cells and their production of cytokines which promotes endometrial growth
Immune dysfunction or deficiency	Prevention of eliminating menstrual debris and promotion of implantation and growth of endometrial lesions
Apoptosis suppression	Survival of endometrial cells by suppression of apoptotic pathways
Genetic	Alteration of cell types to endometriosis lesions
Stem cells	Transformation of haematopoietic, bone marrow or mesenchymal stem cells to endometriosis
Lymphatic, haematogenous metastasis	Spread of endometrial cells by lymphatic or haematogenous vessels
Embryonic cell remnants	Mullerian duct rests, Wolffian duct rests
Multiple factors	Combination of in situ development and endometrial transplantation and implantation
New theory of endometriosis aetiology from primordial germ cells	**The eutopic and ectopic endometrium originating from primordial germ cells**

Germ cells in embryo

Zygote is totipotent, because a single cell has ability to generate all differentiated cells in the entirely embryo. During first weeks of gestation the zygote undergoes to a series of asynchronous holoblastic divisions, increasing the numbers of cells - blastomeres, which form animal pole and vegetative pole. [21-25]

Due to asynchronous division the initial population of blastomeres in the vegetative pole preserves their potency.

The blastomeres are pluripotent, refers to differentiate into 3 germ layers: endoderm, mesoderm and ectoderm. Gastrulation begins with formation of the trilaminar germ disk, the extraembryonic epyblast and hypoblast. [21-25]

In human embryos, the germline epithelium of the indifferent gonads originates from primordial germ cells at the time of gastrulation (at 3 weeks of gestation, equal to Carnegie stages 7 to 9). Initially, the population of primordial germ cells is located in the posterior endoderm that forms the hindgut and yolk sac close to the allantois. At 4–5 weeks of development (Carnegie stages 8–15) the primordial germ cells migrate by amoeboid movement via the hindgut to the dorsolateral gonadal ridges, arriving at the indifferent genital ridges during the 6th week. The indifferent gonad is differentiating into an ovary at 6–8 weeks (Carnegie stages 16–19), and the embryo becomes female. Primordial germ cells subsequently develop into oogonia, but they can enter meiosis or become granulosa cells in primordial follicles. The pathway of primordial germ cell migration has been defined: from the caudal wall of the yolk sac close to the allantois, along the wall of the hindgut and the dorsal mesentery followed by bilateral migration into the genital ridges. [21-25]

There is no evidence of sex-specific differences during primordial germ cells migration in male or female embryos. The maintenance of germ cell potency may be suppressed while they migrate to the somatic gonadal ridges and generate mature sex-specific gametes. [21-25].

New theory of endometriosis origination from primordial germ cells

According to the "New theory of uterovaginal anomalies" (in Chapter III), the eutopic endometrium develops inside of the uterine folds from gonadal ridges, which composed of primordial germ cells.

The uterus develops in the area of intersection between the mesonephral ducts and the gonadal ridges by the fusion of the two (2) uterine folds. The gonadal ridges composed of primordial germ cells derive to the: eutopic endometrium, ovary, ovarian ligament and ligamentum teres uteri. [26, 27]

Germ cells at the gastrulation stage appear among endoderm cells in the wall of the yolk sac close to the allantois. They migrate by amoeboid movement from the hypoblast back to the dorsolateral gonadal ridges along the mesentery of the hindgut (Fig. IV-1).

The hypothetic possibility that the ovary and endometrium derive from the gonadal ridges could be the key point to understanding the aetiologies of external (extragenital) and ovarian endometriosis. For a review see refs. 26-28.

Primordial germ cells derivation in female reproductive organs (Table IV-2):

Germ cells in the ovary differentiate into germline derivatives - oocytes and granulosa cells.

Eutopic endometrium derives from germ cells in crossing area between gonadal ridges with mesonephral ducts.

Ovarian ligamentum proprium and ligamentum teres uteri are remnants of gonadal ridges.

Table IV-2. Primordial germ cells derivation in female reproductive organs. Current views.

Theory	Mechanism
Implantation theory	Retrograde menstruation allowing implantation of endometrial glands in pelvic peritoneum
Coelomic metaplasia	Transformation of peritoneal mesothelium or other cell types into endometrial tissue
Hormonal induction	Oestrogen-driven proliferation of endometrial lesions or metaplasia by hormonal stimulation
Inflammation and oxidative stress	Recruitment of immune cells and their production of cytokines which promotes endometrial growth

Figure IV-1. Primordial germ cells migration pathway. Zygote is totipotent. The blastomeres are pluripotent. Due to asynchronous division the initial population of blastomeres in the vegetative pole preserves their potency. Primordial germ cells are located first at the vegetative pole of blastocyst, then in the hypoblast (yolk sac) to avoid of differentiation signals and maintain the polypotency. After gastrulation the primordial germ cells migrate by amoeboid movement back to the embryo through the peritoneum to the dorsolateral gonadal ridges.

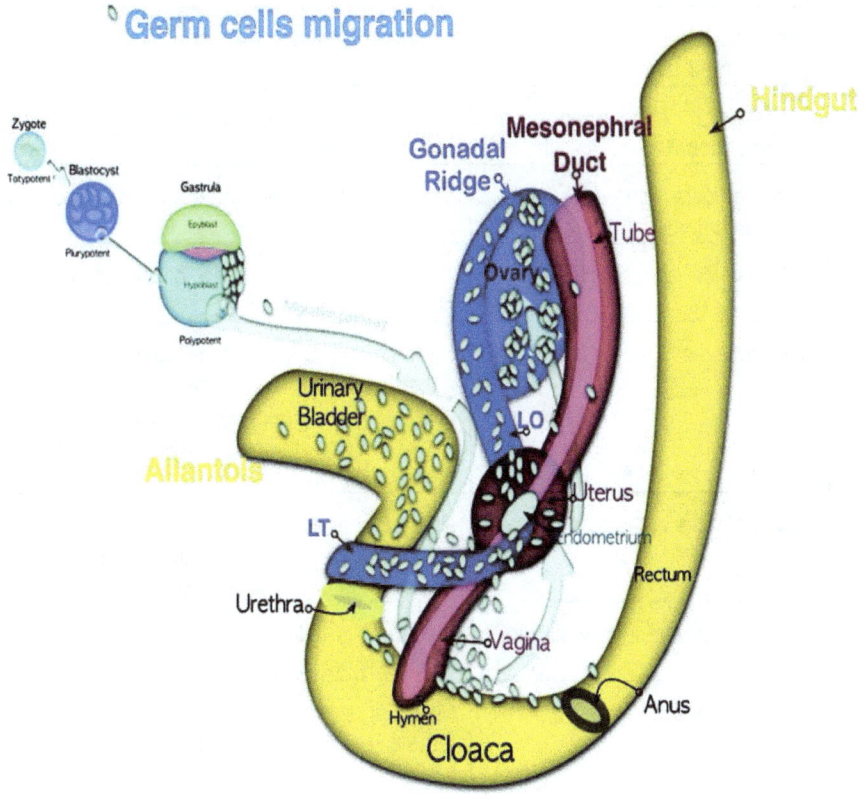

Speculations about the etiology of endometriosis with clinical evidence supporting the new theory

Ovarian endometriosis (Table IV-3) derives by metaplasia of germline epithelium occurring during luteinization (Fig. IV-2).

Table IV-3. New theory of endometriosis aetiology

Endometriosis localization	Derivation
Ovarian cysts	Luteinization of unovulated (unruptured) follicle
Superficial ovarian endometriosis in the cortical layer	On the stigma after ovulation
Extra-genital endometriosis on the peritoneum	Persistence of primordial germ cells on the embryonal pathway
Endometriosis on the utero-sacral ligaments	Most common area of embryonal pathway migration from hindgut
Retrocervical endometriosis	The early pathway area of migration from hindgut
Adenomyosis	Endometrium derives from the intersection of gonadal ridges, containing primordial germ cells, with mesonephral ducts. In the uterine folds there are closer cell-to-cell communications.
Endometriosis in the other area	Primordial germ cells may migrate in the other somatic area from the hypoblast, through the endodermal gut to derivative organs
Endometriosis in urinary bladder	Bladder is derived from the hindgut, especially part of the allantois
Endometriosis in males	Male prostatic glands are analogues of female endometrium. The gubernaculum testis is similar to the uterine broad ligament

Figure IV-2. The luteinization of unovulated follicle (LUF syndrome) in the left ovary: a corpus luteum with endometriotic lesions on the upper pole without ovulatory stigma.

The cases of LUF may be key to understanding infertility in patients with ovarian endometriosis.

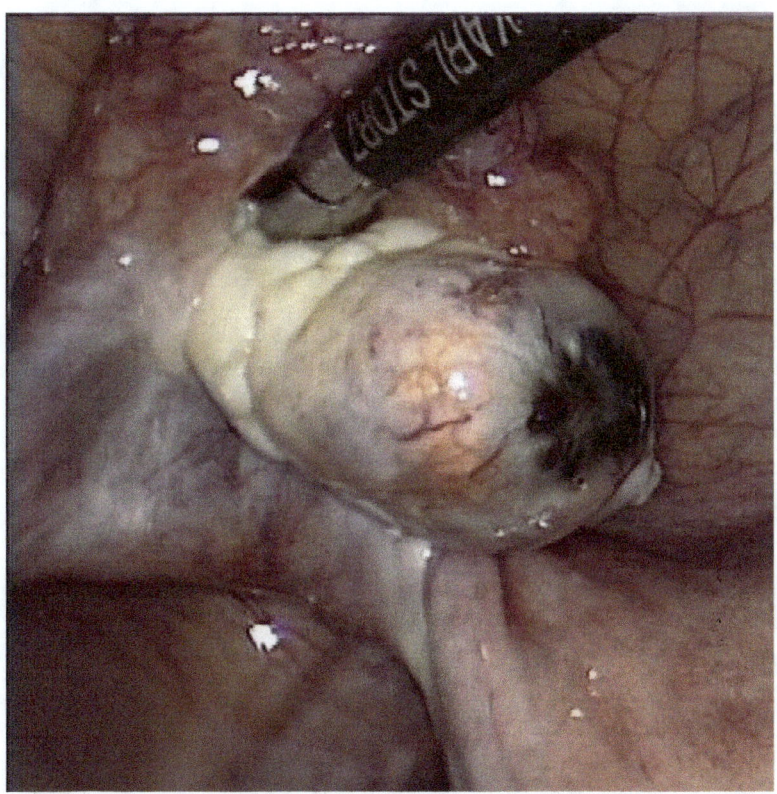

Interesting evidence we found during laparoscopy in patients with primary infertility. In the left ovary, there is a corpus luteum with endometriotic lesions on the upper pole without ovulatory stigma. This is luteinization of the unovulated (or unruptured) follicle (LUF syndrome). Apparently, LUF may be the early stage of aetio-pathological development of the endometriotic cyst.

External endometriosis derives from primordial germ cells during the migration pathway from the yolk sac to the gonadal ridges (Fig. IV-1). The germ cells pathway passes through the recto-vaginal and vesico-uterine surface, which explains the most common localization of ectopic endometrial lesions. Some of the polypotential germ cells fail to reach the ridges and stay in the peritoneal cavity, where they may be transformed into external endometrial heterotopy.

Figure IV-3. Patient with uterovaginal aplasia and non-functioning uterine rudiments had extra-genital endometriosis on the peritoneal surface.

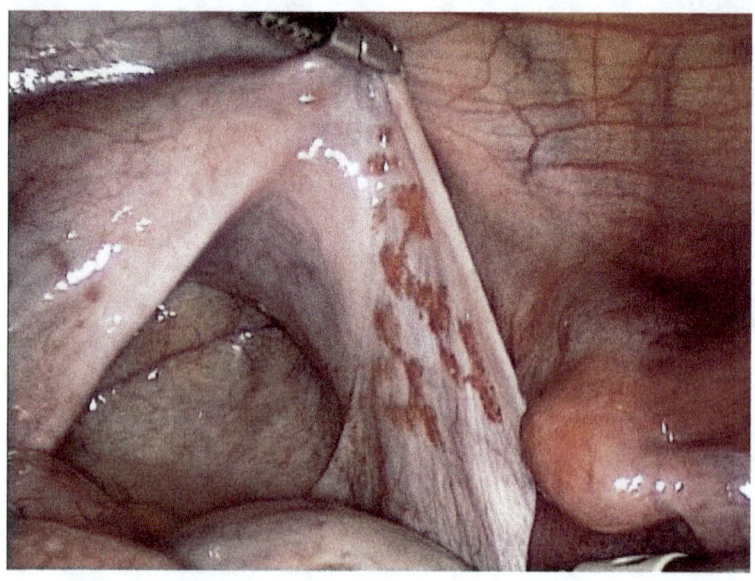

Figure IV-4. The extra-genital endometriosis on the peritoneal surface of the urinary bladder.

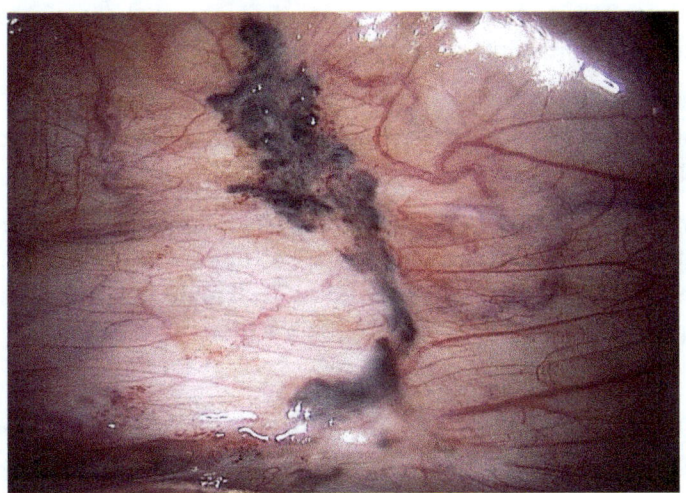

The new theory may explain the presence of endometriosis under the peritoneum in fetuses and females with complete utero-vaginal aplasia (Fig. IV-3) and on the the peritoneal surface of the urinary bladder (Fig. IV-4).

Patient with uterovaginal aplasia (Mayer-Rokitansky-Kuster-Hauser syndrome). The uterine rudiments are non-functional and located at the intersection of the Fallopian tubes with broad and ovarian ligaments. The endometriotic lesions are located superficially on the peritoneum, to the right of the utero-sacral ligament (Fig. IV-3).

The presence of lesions in this area seems to show similarity to the migration pathway (Fig. IV-1).

External endometriosis originates from the primordial germ cells before organogenesis of the reproductive system, and disturbances in germ cell migration to the gonadal ridges can occur.

There are 2 principal processes in uterine organogenesis: intersection of gonadal ridges with mesonephral ducts to form uterine folds with endometrial cavity (eutopic endometrium) and fusion of the both uterine folds together. There are closer cell-to-cell communications in the uterine folds. Polypotential germ cells differentiate and grow into myometrium and endometrial layers.

Endometrial glands may persist at the ovarian ligamentum proprium and ligamentum teres uteri, as they are remnants of the gonadal ridges after complete uterine embryogenesis.

Disorders of these intersections may result in internal endometriosis (adenomyosis). Disorders of uterine fold fusion may result in congenital uterine anomalies. These related processes may explain the high rate of congenital uterine anomalies with concomitant endometriosis.

According to our research, the [26] extra-genital endometriosis was the major concomitant pathology in 46% of patients with various uterovaginal anomalies.

We analyzed the correlation of endometriosis with anomaly type and menstrual outflow obstruction. There were no significant differences between obstructive anomalies (such as partial or complete vaginal aplasia, functional uterine horn) and in non-obstructive symmetric malformations (with uterus duplex, septate uterus).

Histological investigation revealed internal endometriosis in 37% of cases of removed functional uterine rudiments and uterine horns.[26]

Estrogens influence the eutopic and ectopic endometrium survival and proliferation. This effect explains the initiation of manifestation symptoms in females in puberty and progression in reproductive age, especially in females with hyperoestrogenia.

Patients with luteinization of unovulated follicle may also have hyperoestrogenia, which may stimulate progression of extragenital lesions.

Estrogen levels are lower in the male embryo than in the female embryo but are sufficient for the survival of some germ cell populations. Endometriosis in males and 46,XY DSD patients may persist as they migrate at an early stage before sexual differentiation.

Conclusion

According to the new theory, primordial germ cells migrate from hypoblast (yolk sac close to the allantois) to the gonadal ridges. The gonadal ridges which composed of primordial germ cells derive to the: eutopic endometrium, ovary, ovarian ligament and ligamentum teres uteri. There are 2 principal processes in uterine organogenesis: the intersection of gonadal ridges with mesonephral ducts to form the uterine folds with an endometrial cavity and the fusion of the both uterine folds together to form the unicavital (normal) uterus.

In the uterine folds, there are closer cell-to-cell communications, polypotential germ cells differentiate and grow into myometrium and endometrial layers. Some of the polypotential germ cells fail to reach the ridges and stay in the peritoneal cavity, where they may be transforming into external endometrial heterotopies. The main insight in the etiology of endometriosis is polypotential germ cells origin, which may explain its potency, pathogenesis and expansion.

Primordial germ cells initially do not have sex-specific features and have polypotential characteristics during migration. [24]

In female embryo germ cells, those arriving the gonadal ridges give rise to germinal epithelium of the gonads (oocytes, granulosa cells in ovary) and eutopic endometrium.

The ectopic endometrium (endometriosis) originates from primordial germ cells and preserves polypotency (stem cell properties) such as: proliferation, germination, invasion, spread or metastasis by lymphatic and haematogenous pathways.

Germ cell properties of endometrioid lesions should be considered to better understanding the pathogenesis, as they may evolve into a novel target treatment. [29]

The main insight in the etiology of endometriosis is polypotential germ cells origin, which may explain its potency, pathogenesis and expansion.

References

1. Johnson NP, Hummelshoj L, Adamson GD, Keckstein J, Taylor HS, A brao MS, Bush D, Kiesel L, Tamimi R, Sharpe-Timms KL, et al. World Endometriosis Society consensus on the classification of endometriosis. Hum Reprod 2017; 32(2):315-24; https://doi.org/10.1093/humrep/dew293

2. Rogers PA, Adamson GD, Al-Jefout M, Becker CM, D'Hooghe TM, Dunselman GA, Fazleabas A, Giudice LC, Horne AW, Hull ML, et al. WES/WERF consortium for research priorities in endometriosis. Research priorities for endometriosis. Reprod Sci 2017; 24(2):202-26; https://doi.org/10.1177/1933719116654991

3. Ferenczy A. Pathophysiology of adenomyosis. Hum Reprod Update 1998; 4:312-22; PMID:9825847; https://doi.org/10.1093/humupd/4.4.312

4. Knapp VJ. How old is endometriosis? Late 17th and 18th century European descriptions of the disease. Fertil Steril 1999; 72:10-4; PMID:10428141; https://doi.org/10.1016/S0015-0282(99)00196-X

5. Signorile PG, Baldi A. Endometriosis: New concepts in the pathogenesis. Int J Biochem Cell Biol 2010; 42(6):778-80; PMID:20230903; https://doi.org/10.1016/j.biocel.2010.03.008

6. Signorile PG, Baldi F, Bussani R, D'Armiento MR, De Falco M, Boccellino M, Quagliuolo L, Baldi A. New evidence sustaining the presence of endometriosis in the human foetus. Reprod Biomed Online 2010; 21(1):142-7.

7. Signorile PG, Baldi F, Bussani R, D'Armiento MR, DeFalco M, Baldi A. Ectopic endometrium in human fetuses is a common event and sustains the theory of mullerianosis in the pathogenesis of endometriosis, a disease that predisposes to cancer. J Exp Clin Cancer Res 2009; 28:49; https://doi.org/10.1186/1756-9966-28-49

8. DeJolinière JB, Ayoubi JM, Lesec G, Validire P, Goguin A, Gianaroli L, Dubuisson JB, Feki A, Gogusev J. Identification of Displaced Endometrial Glands and Embryonic Duct Remnants in Female Fetal Reproductive Tract: Possible Pathogenetic Role in Endometriotic and Pelvic Neoplastic Processes. Front Physiol 2012; 3:444.

9. Beckman EN, Pintado SO, Leonard GL, Sternberg WH. Endometriosis of the prostate. Am J Surg Pathol 1985; 9(5):374-9; https://doi.org/10.1097/00000478-198505000-00008

10. González RS, Vnencak-Jones CL, Shi C, Fadare O. Endomyometriosis ("Uterus-like mass") in an XY male: case report with molecular confirmation and literature review. Int J Surg Pathol 2014; 22(5):421-6; https://doi.org/10.1177/1066896913501385

11. Sampson J. Peritoneal endometriosis due to the menstrual dissemination of endometrial tissue into the peritoneal cavity. Am J Obstet Gynecol 1927; 14:442-69; https://doi.org/10.1016/S0002-9378(15)30003-X

12. Gruenwald P. Origin of endometriosis from the mesenchyme of the celomic walls. Am JObstetrics Gynecol 1942; 44(3):470-4; https://doi.org/10.1016/S0002-9378(42)90484-8

13. Von Numers. Observations on metaplastic changes in the germinal epithelium of the ovary and on the aetiology of ovarian endometriosis. Acta Obstet Gynecol Scand 1965; 44:107-16; PMID:14299344; https://doi.org/10.3109/00016346509153982

14. Hufnagel D, Li F, Cosar E, Krikun G, Taylor HS. The Role of Stem Cells in the Etiology and Pathophysiology of Endometriosis. Semin Reprod Med 2015; 33(5):333-40; PMID:26375413; https://doi.org/10.1055/s-0035-1564609

15. Sasson E, Taylor HS. Stem cells and the pathogenesis of endometriosis. Ann N Y Acad Sci 2008; 1127:106-15; PMID:18443337; https://doi.org/10.1196/annals.1434.014

16. Jerman LF, Hey-Cunningham AJ. The role of the lymphatic system in endometriosis: a comprehensive review of the literature. Biol Reprod 2015; 92(3):64; PMID:25588508; https://doi.org/10.1095/biolreprod.114.124313

17. Herington JL, Bruner-Tran KL, Lucas JA, Osteen KG. Immune interactions in endometriosis. Expert Rev Clin Immunol 2011; 7(5):611-26; PMID:21895474; https://doi.org/10.1586/eci.11.53

18. Laganà AS, Sturlese E, Retto G, Sofo V, Triolo O. Interplay between misplaced Müllerian-derived stem cells and peritoneal immune dysregulation in the pathogenesis of endometriosis. Obstet Gynecol Int 2013; 2013:527041 ID-527041

19. Sahin AA, Silva EG, Landon G, et al. Endometrial tissue in myometrial vessels not associated with menstruation. Int J Gynecol Pathol 1989; 8:139-46; PMID:2469659; https://doi.org/10.1097/00004347-198906000-00007

20. Sourial S, Tempest N, Hapangama DK. Theories on the pathogenesis of endometriosis. Int J Reprod Med 2014; 2014:179515; PMID:25763392; https://doi.org/10.1155/2014/179515

21. Bukovsky A. Ovarian Stem Cell Niche and Follicular Renewal in Mammals. Anat Rec 2011; 294(8):1284-306; https://doi.org/10.1002/ar.21422

22. Heeren AM, He N, de Souza AF, Goercharn-Ramlal A, van Iperen L, Roost MS, Gomes Fernandes MM, van der Westerlaken LA, Chuva de Sousa Lopes SM. On the development of extragonadal and gonadal human germ cells. Biol Open 2016; 5(2):185-94; PMID:26834021; https://doi.org/10.1242/bio.013847

23. Seydoux G, Braun RE. Pathway to totipotency: lessons from germ cells. Cell 2006; 127(5):891-904; PMID:17129777; https://doi.org/10.1016/j.cell.2006.11.016

24. Wear HM, McPike MJ, Watanabe KH. From primordial germ cells to primordial follicles: a review and visual representation of early ovarian development in mice. J Ovarian Res 2016; 9;36; PMID:27329176; https://doi.org/10.1186/s13048-016-0246-7

25. Hill MA. UNSW Embryology 2017. Primordial Germ Cell Migration Movie. https://embryology.med.unsw.edu.au/embryology/index.php/Primordial_Germ_Cell_Migration_Movie [Google Scholar]

26. Makiyan Z. New theory of uterovaginal embryogenesis. Organogenesis 2016; 12(1):33-41; PMID:26900909; https://doi.org/10.1080/15476278.2016.1145317

27. Makiyan Z. Studies of gonadal sex differentiation. Organogenesis 2016; 12(1):42-51; PMID:26950283; https://doi.org/10.1080/15476278.2016.1145318

28. Makiyan Z. Systematization of ambiguous genitalia. Organogenesis 2016; 12(4):169-82; PMID:27391116; https://doi.org/10.1080/15476278.2016.1210749

29. Binda MM, Donnez J, Dolmans MM. Targeting mast cells: a new way to treat endometriosis. Expert Opin Ther Targets 2017; 21(1):67-75; PMID:27841046; https://doi.org/10.1080/14728222.2017.1260548

V. AMBIGUOUS EXTERNAL GENITALIA

Introduction

Human organogenesis begins in the third week of gestation when the paraxial mesoderm organizes into segments, known as somitomeres (somites). During that period, the three germ layers, consisting of the ectoderm, the mesoderm, and the endoderm, give rise to a number of specific tissues and organs. [1]

The first somites appear in the cephalic region of the embryo at approximately the 20th day of development, and their formation proceeds cephalo-caudally at a rate of approximately three pairs per day. At the end of the fifth week, the embryo has 42-44 pairs of somites; these consist of 4 occipital, 8 cervical, 12 thoracic, 5 lumbar, 5 sacral, and 8 to 10 coccygeal pairs. [1]

Each somitomere consists of mesodermal cells arranged in concentric whorls around the centre of the unit. Somites give rise to the following 5 components: the myotome (segmental muscle component), the sclerotome (cartilage and bone component), and the dermatome (forms the skin of the back). All of these tissues are supporting tissues of the body; each myotome and dermatome retains its own innervation and vascularization from its originating segments, and these form the neurotome and angiotome, respectively. [1, 2]

The vertebral column and ribs retain segmental structure. They develop from the sclerotome compartments of the somites, and they join in the ventral body wall. Each segment includes all of the following 5 components: a vertebra connected to a rib (sclerotome), with intercostal muscles (myotome) beneath, and its own nerve (neurotome) and vessels (angiotome), covered in skin (dermatome). The first occipital and the last five to seven coccygeal somites later disappear, while the remaining somites form the axial skeleton. [1]

Initially, the genital system consists of (1) gonads or primitive sex glands, (2) genital ducts and (3) indifferent external genitalia. All three components go through indifferent stages, after which they develop following male or female pathways. [1-5].

The organogenesis of the external genitalia proceeds from the third to the 12th weeks of embryonic development. In the third week of development, mesenchymal cells originating around the primitive streak migrate to the cloacal membrane to form a pair of slightly elevated cloacal folds.
Cranially of the cloacal membrane, the folds unite to form the genital tubercle. Caudally, the folds are subdivided into urethral (anterior) and anal (posterior). Meanwhile, another pair of elevations, the genital swellings, becomes visible on each side of the urethral folds. These swellings later form the scrotal buds (in males) and the labia majora (in females).
The external genitalia in both sexes develop from the genital tubercle, genital swellings, and genital folds. At the end of the sixth week, the genital tubercle is indistinguishable between male and female. [1]

The indifferent duct system and external genitalia develop under the influence of hormones.

In males, the SRY gene on the Y chromosome produces testes-determining factor and regulates male sexual development. Testosterone produced by Leydig cells in the testes stimulates development of the mesonephric ducts into the vas deferens and epididymis. Dihydrotestosterone stimulates development of the male genitalia (virilization), consisting of the penis, scrotum, and prostate. The genital swellings become the scrotum, and the genital tubercle elongates to form the penis (phallus) and the penile urethra, which terminates in the glans penis. The prostate forms in the walls of the urogenital sinus. [1-5].

In the absence or inactivity of androgens, the foetus remains in the indifferent stages and becomes phenotypically female. Estrogens stimulate development of the external genitalia in females. In females, the genital tubercle becomes the clitoris, the genital swellings become the labia majora, and the genital folds become the labia minora. The genital tubercle elongates slightly and forms the clitoris, which is larger than that in the male during the early stages of development. The urethral fold does not fuse, as in the male embryo, and develops into the labia minora. Genital swellings enlarge and form the labia majora. The urogenital groove is open and forms the vestibulum vaginae. [1-6].

Abnormal androgen effects during embryogenesis may cause persistence on between developmental stages, which may result in the foetus clinically presenting as intersexual (disorders of sex development), or it could result in the foetus developing and being assigned female sex at birth. For a review, see refs. [7-16].

Disorders of sex development (DSD) or intersexuality (ambiguity) are present in 0.018% (1.8 per 10,000 live births) of newborns, and the incidence of 46,XY DSD is estimated at 1 in 20,000 live male births. More than 90% of 46,XX patients (congenital adrenal hyperplasia) and 46,XY DSD patients (androgen insensitivity syndrome, testicle dysgenesis) are assigned as females and require for feminizing plasty. [7, 8]

Feminizing genital surgery is considered in cases of severe virilization (Prader degree of III-V) and should be performed with introitoplasty of the common urogenital sinus. [9-18].

Surgical procedures should be anatomically based to preserve the innervation of the clitoris, which possesses erogenous sensation and orgasmic function. [17]

Management of intersex disorders has been addressed in clinical guidelines, but appropriate surgical corrections have not been established in a standardized fashion for gynaecological practice. [9-14]

Materials and methods

All individuals received an assignment of female gender after clinical examination, karyotyping, ultrasonography, MRI, laparoscopy, studies of gonadal morphology, and hormonal measurement.

Surgical correction was performed according to the European Consensus, Chicago Consensus (2006, 2009, 2018) and the UK Guidance (2011) on management of Disorders of Sexual Development (DSD). For a review, see refs. 9-14.

Adnexectomy recommended in SRY-positive female patients with androgen insensitivity syndrome (AIS); 46,XY gonadal dysgenesis, and ovotesticular DSD, to prevent the development of malignancy in adulthood. Gonadal biopsy in SRY negative patients allow for verification of ovarian dysgenesis (45,X/46,XX) or streak-gonads with X-monosomy and mosaicism. Feminizing surgery includes clitororeduction and introitoplasty, which are intended to provide sexual function, retain erogenous sensitivity and achieve a satisfactory cosmetic result. [9-14]

The investigation of gonadal morphology among patients with DSD was published in "Studies of gonadal sex differentiation". [19]

Uterovaginal anomalies were researched in the "New theory of uterovaginal embryogenesis". [20]

The degree of external genitalia virilization was estimated by Prader classification stages I-V (tab. 2). [15, 16]

Clitoreduction was performed for patients with severe virilization (Prader degrees III–V). [9-14]

Results

Differential diagnosis of patients with DSD involves the investigation of karyotype, gonadal morphology, internal genital anatomy and degree of external genital virilization, which guides surgical treatment.

Prader's classification of ambiguous external genitalia includes the following (tab. V-2):

- Prader stage 0 corresponds to females with normal external genitalia. This includes females with 45,X and 45,X/46,XX Turner syndrome and those with a complete form of 46,XY gonadal dysgenesis and androgen insensitivity syndromes (AIS) who present with feminine external genitalia (Prader stage 0).
- Prader stage I is characterized by a slightly enlarged clitoris. Prader I may be regarded as a common condition present in the general female population.
- Prader stage II distinguishes a mild degree of virilization and does not require surgical correction.
- Prader stage III-V is recognized as ambiguous genitalia or intersex DSD. Patients with ambiguous genitalia (Prader degree III-V) undergo feminizing genitoplasty according to the European Consensus recommendations.
- Prader VI stage indicates a normal male presentation with typical external genitalia and normal testes in the scrotum.

First-line surgery is performed for patients with 46,XY gonadal dysgenesis, testicular feminization syndrome and ovotesticular DSD: laparoscopic adnexectomy to remove the testicular tissue or rudimentary gonads.

Feminizing surgery of the external genitalia was performed in cases with Prader degree III-V, and some of them had V degree of masculinization.

Feminizing surgery includes clitororeduction and introitoplasty, which are intended to retain erogenous sensitivity and achieve a satisfactory cosmetic result.

The clitoris is innervated by sensory nerves that pass within the nervus dorsalis clitoridis and the nervus pudendalis originating from S2-S5 segments. Surgical incision of the clitoral glans and corpora cavernosa may risk damaging the innervation, which disturbs the erogenous sensation essential for orgasm. Problems related with clitoroplasty are decreased sexual sensitivity, loss of clitoral tissue, and cosmetic issues. The surgical procedure of clitororeduction relies anatomically on the precise incision of the corpora cavernosa and preservation of innervation of the glans clitoris.

The modified clitororeduction, as opposed to clitorectomia, is performed by resection of the corpora cavernosa and preservation of the glans clitoridis on the dorsal and ventral neurovascular bundles (Fig. V-1, 2).

The surgical operation stages proceed as follows. A semilunar incision is made around the glans clitoridis at a distance of 5-7 mm. The isolated clitoral shaft (body) is completely separated before the pubic bone. On the sides of the clitoris shaft, longitudinally lateral cuts of Buck's fascia and the tunica albuginea are made. The corpora cavernosa is sharply mobilized and separated from the glans clitoris until bifurcation of the crura clitoridis, and it is cut off just above of symphysis (pubic bone). The isolated dorsal and ventral neurovascular bundle is mobilized and preserved, and the connection to the glans clitoridis is maintained. The glans clitoris on the dorsal neurovascular bundle is connected and sutured with the cult of the resected corpora cavernosa. The ventral sheaf is underlined on the vestibulum vaginae. The capuche is formed above the glans clitoris and around the pudendal labia minora from prepuceal skin.

In patients with a common urogenital sinus, was performed the Y-shape introitoplasty. Briefly, the surgery began with vertical cutting of the urogenital orificium (opening) down to the perineum. Then, the internal mucosa was turned outwards, circumcised along the sides and sewed edge-to-edge with the skin incision. The widely shaped vaginal introitus was formed (Fig. V-4a, b).

Postoperative examination showed positive cosmetic results, feminine-appearing genitalia and preservation of the erogenous sensibility of the clitoris, vestibulum vaginae and labia minora.

The second-line surgery consists of the creation of a neovagina, and this is performed for patients with Turner syndrome, AIS, incomplete 46,XY gonadal dysgenesis, and ovotesticular DSD with uterovaginal aplasia.

Systematization of the clinical features and anatomy of the external genitalia of female patients with DSD is presented in table V-1, including some clinico-anatomical differences in DSD variants.

The complete diagnosis of patterns of intersex disorders is provided by investigation of the karyotype, gonadal morphology, internal genital anatomy (tab. V-1), with indication of external genital virilization stages by Prader (tab. V-2).

The major groups of DSD females described below in the sequence, as they specified in the table V-1:

- ✓ 46,XX karyotype – congenital adrenal hyperplasia;
- ✓ X chromosome monosomy in the 3 variants of Turner syndrome;
- ✓ 46,XY karyotype - androgen insensitivity syndrome and gonadal dysgenesis;
- ✓ Ovotesticular DSD.

Some clinical cases of ambiguity have presented as most demonstrative.

Patients with congenital adrenal hyperplasia (CAH) have normal ovaries, uterus and vagina.

The 11% of patients had uterovaginal malformations: septate uterus and underwent hysteroresection, and duplicated uterus and vagina.

The 9% of patients with ambiguous external genitalia had a clitoris larger than 5-6 cm, and 2% of patients had Prader degree V masculinization.

Surgical treatment includes clitororeduction and introitoplasty.

Clinical case. Patient 1, 18 years aged (Fig. V-1a). External genitalia was ambiguous, corresponds to Prader stage III. She had congenital uterine anomaly: subseptate uterus with normal vagina.

Hormonal measurement before gonadectomy revealed severe hyperandrogenia: LG – 31.7↑ (3.0-10.0) Eq/l, FSH - 29↑ (3.0-8.0) Eq/l, Prl – 297 (120-500) mEq/l, Cortisol - 625 (200-500) nml/l, DHEAS – 22.8 (0.9-11.7) mcml/l, E2 – 62 (150-480) nml/l, 17-OHP – 143 (6-16) nml/l, T – 25,4↑ (1.0-2.5) nml/l.

Figure V-1. Congenital adrenal hyperplasia. Prader stage III.

Figure V-1a. External genitalia before operation. Clitoromegaly and sinus urogenitalis resulted of incomplete posterior labial fusion.

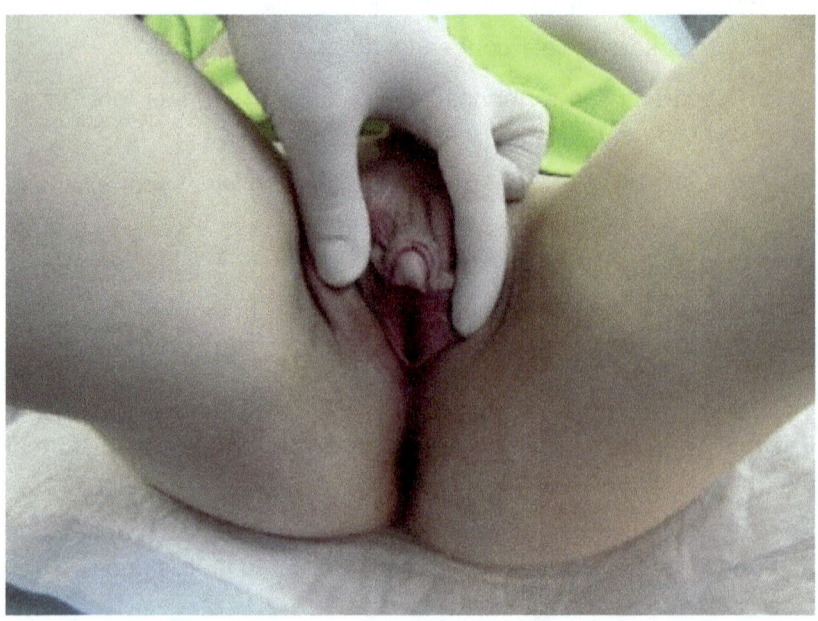

Surgical treatment includes clitororeduction and introitoplasty (Fig. 1-B). Hysteroresectoscopic metroplasy also performed.

Figure V-1b. External genitalia after clitororeduction and introitoplasty.

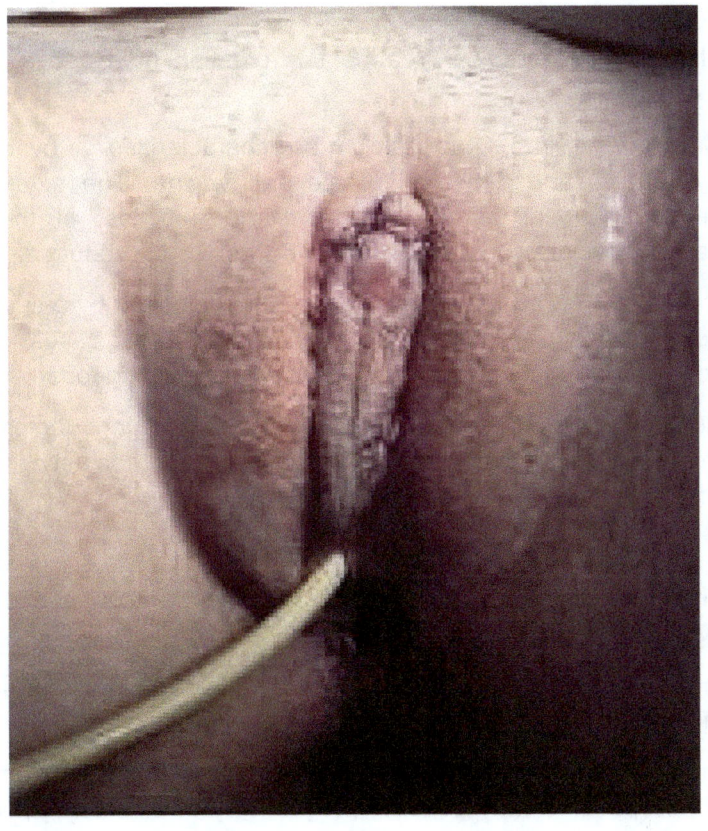

Turner syndrome is characterized by X chromosome monosomy and has 3 distinct forms, for which surgical treatment differs.

- The classical form (45,X) is characterized by fibrous streak in the gonads and persistence of Mullerian ducts derivates (PMDS). The external genitalia appear female (Prader stage 0).

  The indicated surgical treatment is creation of a neovagina (colpopoesis) only.

- Cases of 45,X/46,XX mosaicism are characterized by ovarian dysgenesis and a normal uterus and vagina. The external genitalia appear female (Prader stage 0). Most of these patients ovulate and may be fertile. Surgery is not required.

- Cases of 45,X/46,XY mosaicism are characterized by a streak gonad or streak testes (or ovotestis). These cases are considered PMDS. The external genitalia are ambiguous.

  Surgical treatment consists of laparoscopy and gonadectomy, feminizing genitoplasty (clitororeduction and introitoplasty), and colpopoesis.

The 46,XY gonadal (testicle) dysgenesis may present in one of two forms.

- In the complete form, the uterus and vagina are present, and the external genitalia appear female (Prader stage 0).

  Surgical treatment consists of laparoscopy and gonadectomy. These patients may become pregnant by in vitro fertilization (IVF) using donor oocytes.

- The incomplete form presented of PMDS (or uterus and vagina). The external genitalia are ambiguous.

Surgical treatment consists of laparoscopy and gonadectomy, feminizing genitoplasty (clitororeduction and introitoplasty), and colpopoesis.

Clinical case. Patient 2, 14 years aged (Fig. V-2a). She has normal shaped uterus and vagina. Severe clitoromegaly (approximately 5-6 sm), that corresponds to Prader III–IV stages. Vaginal vestibulum had normal orificium (opening).

Hormonal measurement before gonadectomy: LG – 40.7↑ (3.0-10.0) Eq/l, FSH - 109↑ (3.0-8.0) Eq/l, Prl – 297 (120-500) mEq/l, Cortisol - 425 (200-500) nmi/l, DHEAS – 6.3 (0.9-11.7) mcml/l, E2 – 273 (150-480) nml/l, 17-OHP – 4.3 (6-16) nml/l, T – 6.5↑ (1.0-2.5) nml/l.

Surgery treatment: gonadectomy and clitoreduction was performed. On the Fig.2-B presented the operation stage of resection of the corpora cavernosa with preserving the glans clitoridis connected with dorsal and ventral neurovascular bundles.

The external genitalia in 3 week after operation (Fig. 2-C)

Clinical case. Patient 3, 19 years aged. She was assigned as a male newborn, but in 17 years reassigned to female gender. Gonads appear as streak-testes, located in the abdomen and removed laparoscopically. Uterus and vagina are absent.

Hormonal measurement before gonadectomy revealed hypergonadotropic hypogonadism, low level of androgens: LG – 13.8↑ (3.0-10.0) Eq/l, FSH – 29.2↑ (3.0-8.0) Eq/l, Prl – 140 (120-500) mEq/l, Cortisol - 245 (200-500) nmi/l, DHEAS – 1.6 (0.9-11.7) mcml/l, E2 – 65.6↓ (150-480) nml/l, 17-OHP – 5.0↓ (6-16) nml/l, T – 0.37↓ (1.0-2.5) nml/l.

Figure V-2. 46,XY gonadal (testicle) dysgenesis, incomplete form.
Figure V-2a: External genital view before operation. Clitoromegaly (appr. 5-6 sm), corresponds to Prader stage III-IV. The vagina introitus normal corresponds to Prader 0 (arrow).

Figure V-2b: The stage of clitororeduction: separated glans clitoris connected with dorsal (N) and ventral (V) neurovascular bundles; corpora cavernosa clitoridis (V).

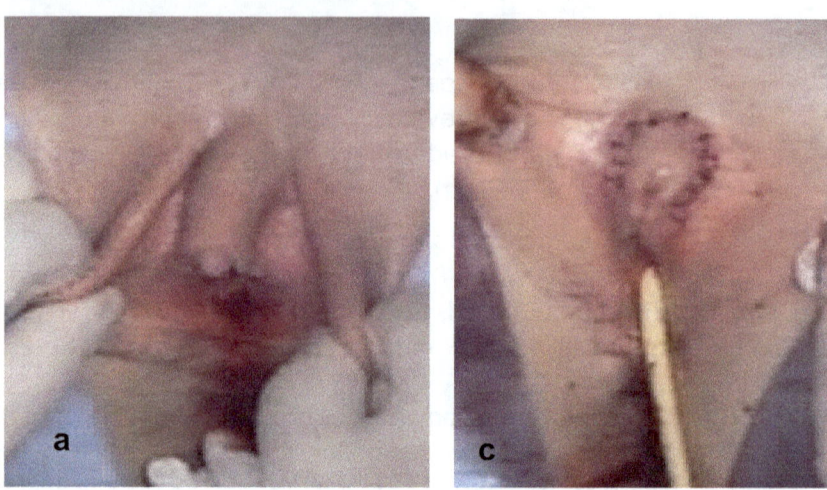

Figure V-2c, d: The external genitalia after clitororeduction by recection of corpora cavernosa, in 3 week after operation.

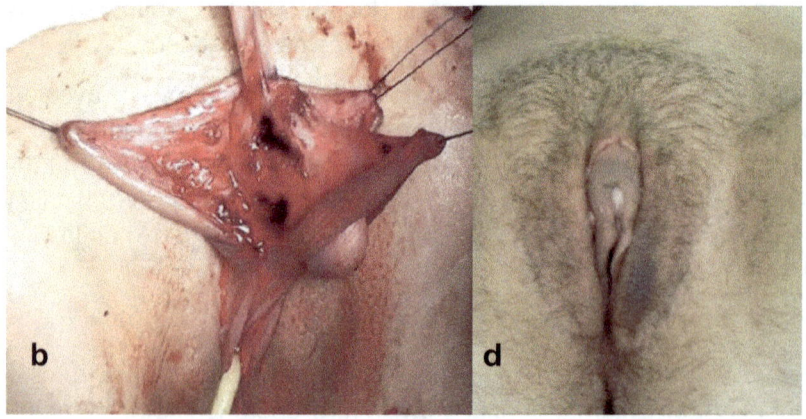

External genitalia have male phenotype with micropenis. Complete fusion of the labial folds persisted, the urogenital sinus transforming to the penile urethra, with single orifice at the top of glans penis. This stage corresponds to Prader V degree (Fig. V-3).
First line surgery performed gonadectomy and introitoplasty; second line – creation of neovagina.

Figure V-3. 46,XY gonadal (testicle) dysgenesis. External genitalia corresponds to Prader stage V. Micropenis and complete labial fusion to penile (masculine) urethra.

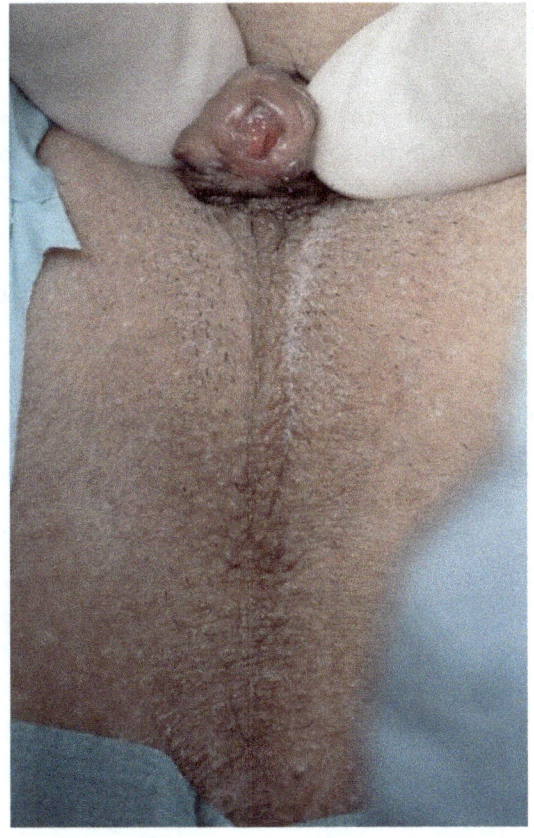

Androgen insensitivity syndrome may present in one of two forms.

> ➢ The complete form presented of rudimental structures of PMDS (Fallopian tubes and uterine rudiments), and the external genitalia appear female (Prader stage 0).
>
> Surgical treatment consists of laparoscopy, gonadectomy, and colpopoesis.
>
> ➢ The incomplete form presented of rudimental structures of PMDS, and the external genitalia appear ambiguous.
>
> Surgical treatment consists of laparoscopy, gonadectomy, feminizing genitoplasty, and colpopoesis.

Clinical case. Patient 4, 14 years aged. Androgen insensitivity syndrome, incomplete form. Corresponds to Prader stage IV. The clitororeduction was performed before (Fig. V-4a). The urogenital sinus opens near of the base clitoris. The Y-shaped introitoplasty realized on the second line (Fig. V-4b, c).

The complete diagnosis, by new systematization, which is proposed in Chapter VI:

Karyotype 46,XY. [Gonadal morphology] Testis. [Internal anatomy] Unicavital terus and vagina. [Viriliztion degree] Prader III.

Surgical treatment performed according to definition: gonadectomy, clitororeduction and Y-shaped introitoplasty.

Figure V-4. Androgen insensitivity syndrome, incomplete form.
Figure V-4a: External genital view after clitororeduction. The urogenital sinus opens near of the base clitoris.

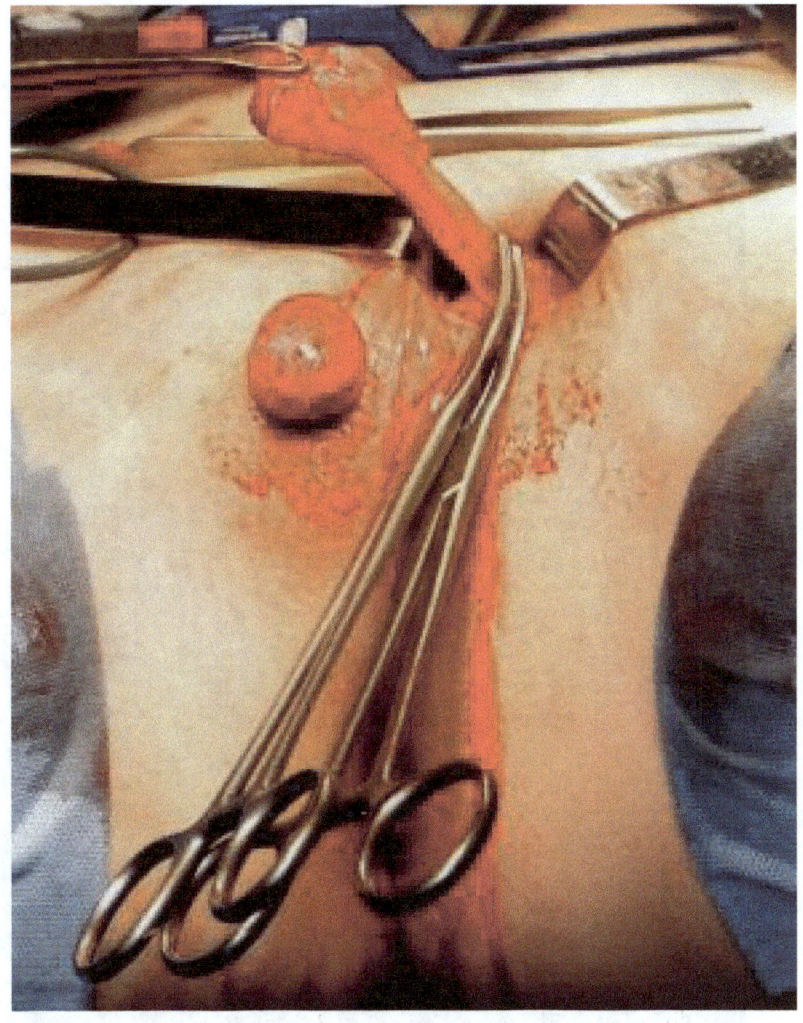

Figure V-4b: The Y-shaped introitoplasty. The vertical cutting of the urogenital sinus opens the orificium. The internal mucosa was turned outwards, and located edge-to-edge with the skin incision before suturing. The widely shaped vaginal introitus was formed.

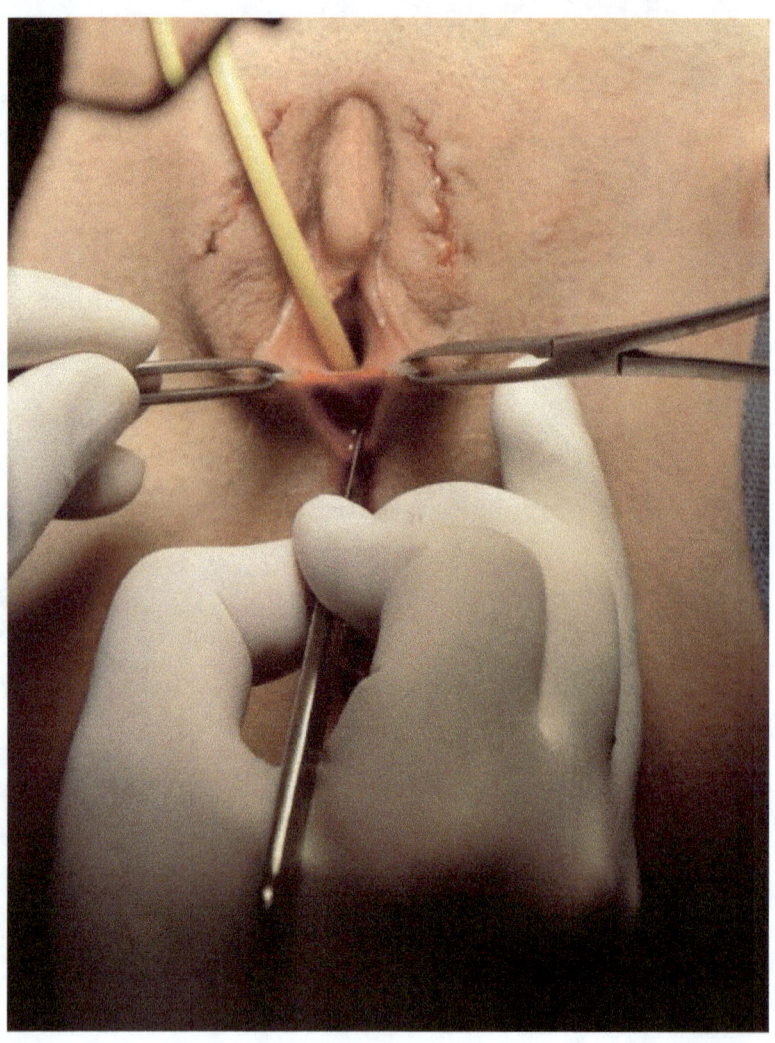

Figure V-4c: The Y-shaped introitoplasty. The internal mucosa was turned outwards, and located edge-to-edge with the skin incision before suturing. The widely shaped vaginal introitus was formed.

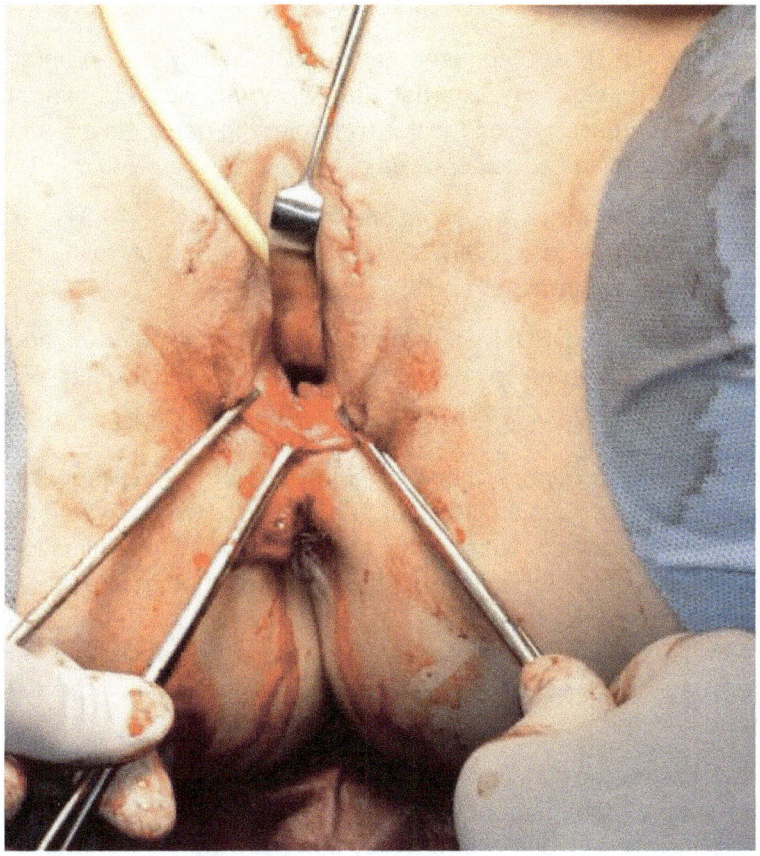

The key differences between AIS and 46,XY gonadal dysgenesis are that AIS has only rudimental PMDS, while some patients with testicle dysgenesis have a uterus and vagina and thus may become pregnant (by IVF with donor oocytes). The external genitalia in both cases may be female or ambiguous.

Ovotesticular DSD is diagnosed by various karyotype and has PMDS with ambiguous external genitalia. Surgical treatment consists of laparoscopy, gonadectomy, feminizing genitoplasty, and creation of a neovagina (colpopoesis).

Ultrasound and MRI investigations revealed the 10.3% of intersexual patients (especially those with CAH) had uterovaginal anomalies that required metroplasty.

Systematization of DSD by distinguishing gonadal, internal and external genital morphology should facilitate differential diagnosis and the choice of an appropriate surgical correction.

The validity of the current classification systems of female genital malformations has been challenged. The proposed VCUAM (vagina cervix uterus adnex - associated malformations) classification makes it possible to estimate the anatomy of pathological uterovaginal malformations. [21, 22] The structure of the system used to reflect oncologic tumours in the TNM classification served as the basis for establishing a new classification of genital malformations. [22]

We encourage the use of the DSD systematization to guide diagnosis and management in gynaecological practice. Applying the "karyotype-gonadal morphology-internal genital anatomy-external genital virilization stages" facilitates diagnosis and appropriate surgical management. This systematization may be extended horizontally to include "reproduction" and "hormonal treatment", and it may be continued vertically to describe new atypical anomalies (tab. V-2, tab. VI-1).

Table V-1. Classification of ambiguous external genitalia by Prader stages.

Prader stages	Clitoromegally	Introitus	Operation
0 stage	Female phenotype, normal clitoris	Normal vestibulum vaginae and labia minora	
I stage	Slightly enlarged clitoris	Normal vaginal orifice	
II stage	Mild enlarged cliitoris	Slightly reduced vaginal orifice and posterior labial fusion. The vagina and urethra open into a funnel-shaped urogenital sinus.	Introitoplasty
III stage	Clitoromegaly	Incomplete posterior fusion of the labia minora. The vagina and urethra share a single opening in the urogenital sinus.	Clitororeduction, introitoplasy
IV stage	Clitoromegaly appears as male phallus	Complete posterior fusion of the labia minora. The urogenital sinus opens near of the base clitoris.	Clitororeduction, introitoplasy
V stage	Male phenotype due to penile transformation (male phallus)	Complete fusion of the labial folds. The urogenital sinus transforming to penile urethra, has single orifice at the glans penis. The normally formed scrotum empty.	Clitororeduction, introitoplasy

Table V-2. Example of Unified Systematization for Intersexual Disorders (DSD)

\multicolumn{6}{c}{Systematization of Intersex Disorders}					
Nosology	Karyotype	Gonadal morphology	Internal genital anatomy	External genital anatomy	Surgical treatment
Congenital adrenal hyperplasia	46,XX	ovary	normal uterus and vagina	ambiguous genitalia	feminizing plasty: clitororeduction, introitoplasty
Turner syndrome (45,X)	45,X	fibrous streak gonad	PMDS	female	colpopoesis
Turner syndrome (45,X/46,XX)	45,X/46,XX	ovarian dysgenesis	normal uterus and vagina	female	laparoscopy gonadal biopsy
Turner syndrome (45,X/46,XY)	45,X/46,XY	fibrous streak, testicular dysgenesis, ovotestis	PMDS	ambiguous genitalia	laparoscopy gonadectomy; feminizing plasty, colpopoesis
46,XY gonadal dysgenesis, incomplete form	46,XY	testicular dysgenesis	PMDS, hypoplastic uterus	ambiguous genitalia	Laparoscopy gonadectomy; feminizing plasty, colpopoesis
46,XY gonadal dysgenesis, complete form	46,XY	testicular dysgenesis	hypoplastic uterus and vagina	female	laparoscopy gonadectomy
Androgen insensitivity syndrome, complete form	46,XY	testicles	PMDS	female	laparoscopy gonadectomy, colpopoesis
Androgen insensitivity syndrome, incomplete form	46,XY	testicles	PMDS	ambiguous genitalia	laparoscopy gonadectomy; feminizing plasty, colpopoesis
Ovotesticular DSD	46,XY 46,XX/46,XY	ovotestis	PMDS	ambiguous genitalia	laparoscopy gonadectomy; feminizing plasty, colpopoesis

Discussion

Sex assignment in newborns depends on the anatomy of the external genitalia, despite this stage being the final stage in embryogenesis.

Systematization of intersex disorders distinguishes the karyotype, gonadal morphology, and genital anatomy to provide a differential diagnosis and guide appropriate surgical management (tab. V-1).

Patients with CAH, Turner syndrome (45,X/46,XX) and some of 46,XY gonadal (testicle) dysgenesis have uterus and vagina (tab. V-1).

The precise ultrasound (or MRI) investigations of internal organ's anatomy important for intersexual females, because 10.3% of them had uterovaginal anomalies, required additional surgical correction.

The estimation of external genital virilization degree carried out by Prader stages in all patients (tab. V-2). The modified feminizing clitoroplasty with preservation of the dorsal and ventral neurovascular bundles to retain erogenous sensitivity was performed only in females with severe virilization degree, according to Prader stages III-V.

The outgrowth of the genital tubercle and the fusion of the urethral fold proceed in an ordered fashion.

In presented cases of ambiguity in 46,XY gonadal (testicle) dysgenesis revealed discordance between virilization degree between clitoris size and urogenital fusion of labial fold. For example, Patient 2 (Fig. V-2a) has severe clitoromegaly and normal vaginal opening; but Patient 3 (Fig. V-3) has micropenis (looks like normal clitoris) and complete labial fusion to penile (masculine) urethra. These cases demonstrate the deviations of external organs development pathways, due to different derivations, influences of growth factors and receptors.

During feminizing surgery detected some nuances: the branches of clitoris located deep inside in the labial folds and surround of vestibulum vaginae.

Androgens and estrogens are typically associated with sexual differentiation of the genitalia and secondary sex characters.

Alfred Jost's model of sexual differentiation considers that in the absence or inactivity of androgen, the foetus remains in the indifferent stages and becomes phenotypically female (independently of karyotype or gonadal morphology).3

Androgens (testosterone and dihydrotestosterone) and estradiol signal by means of androgen receptors (AR) and estrogen receptors (ERa and ERb), respectively. While good progress has been made in identifying the molecules involved in the initiation of limb budding, the initiation of genital outgrowth is not well understood. An interaction between the endoderm and the ectoderm at the cloacal membrane may be an important step in induction of budding. [5, 6, 24-26]

Longstanding dogma is that the sexually indifferent genital tubercle is masculinized by androgens and that feminization is a default state that occurs in the absence of androgen activity, though recent studies of ER mutants have falsified this hypothesis. [5]

Thus, in the absence of ERa activity, female external genitalia are partially masculinized, suggesting that estrogen is required for inhibition of clitoral growth in females. This raises the intriguing possibility that basal levels of androgen in females can lead to masculinization of the genital tubercle, and estrogen is required to counter the influence of androgen. [5, 6, 26, 27]

Mutations in the androgen receptor (as in the testicular feminization or Tfm mutation), by contrast, cause feminization of the external genitalia, such that Tfm mutant male genitalia are indistinguishable from female genitalia. [26]

Mutations in the gene that encodes 5a-reductase 2, which converts testosterone to dihydrotestosterone, also disrupt masculinization of the genital tubercle and cause defects ranging from hypospadias and micropenis to complete feminization of the external genitalia. [8, 27]

Together, these results suggest that the balance of androgens to estrogen is a critical factor in determining sexual differentiation of the genitalia.

Martin Cohn reported, that surgical manipulations of the genital tubercle identified cell populations with functions that appear to be analogous to the apical ectodermal ridge (AER). [5]

Petiot et al. showed that FgfR2, which is essential for urethral tube closure, contains an androgen response element in its promoter, and antagonism of AR results in down-regulation of FgfR2 in the urethral plate and prepuce. [25]

Intersexuality (ambiguity) in 46,XY patients results from disruptors in the pathways of sex steroid hormones and receptors; in 46,XX females this arises from the effects of excess androgen. These processes develop differently but result in the same ambiguity.
Systematic clinical analysis and a literature review revealed the following questions:

- From where does the genital tubercle originate?

- According to the current view, the indifferent genital tubercle originates from mesenchymal tissue, but mesenchymal cells are arranged across the embryonal body and do not have specific androgen receptors.

- Why do androgens cause virilization, and particularly, why does this hormonal influence promote the outgrowth and elongation of the genital tubercle? (Fig. V-5, Fig. V-6)

Figure V-5. The indifferent genital tubercle of female human embryo on Carnegie stage 20 (week 8, 51 - 53 days, 18 - 22 mm), gestational age - week 10.

Sagittal histology. Retrived from UNSW Embryology: https://embryology.med.unsw.edu.au/embryology/images/a/a8/K15818_Stage_20_sagittal_02.jpg

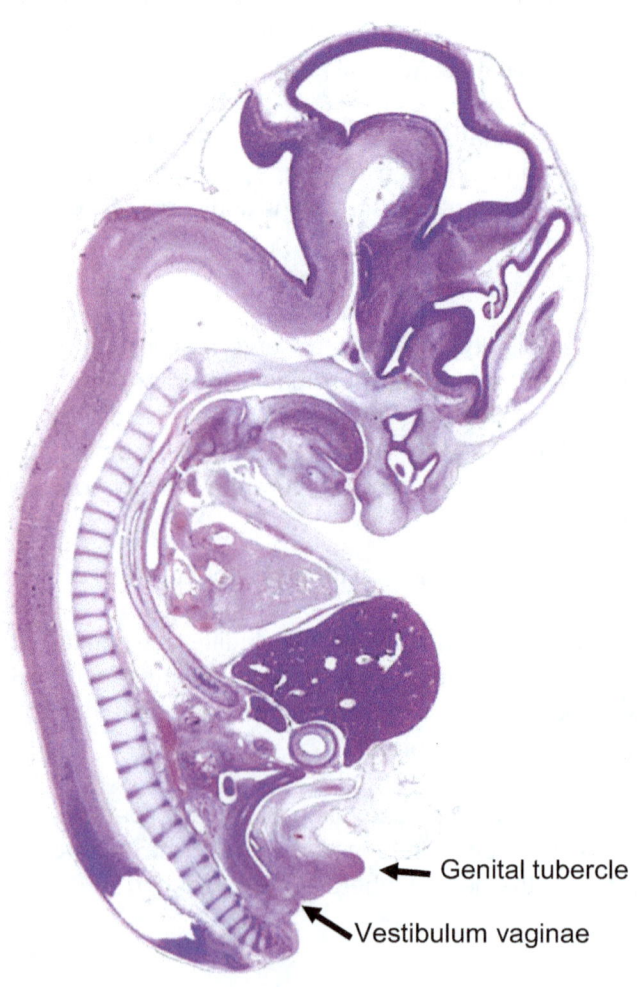

Figure V-6. Genital tubercle (phallus) and penile urethra in a male human embryo on Carnegie stage 22 (week 8, 54 - 56 days, 23 - 28 mm), gestational age week 10.

Serial section. Retrived from UNSW Embryology: https://embryology.med.unsw.edu.au/embryology/index.php/Carnegie_stage_22#/media/File:Stage_22_image_048.jpg

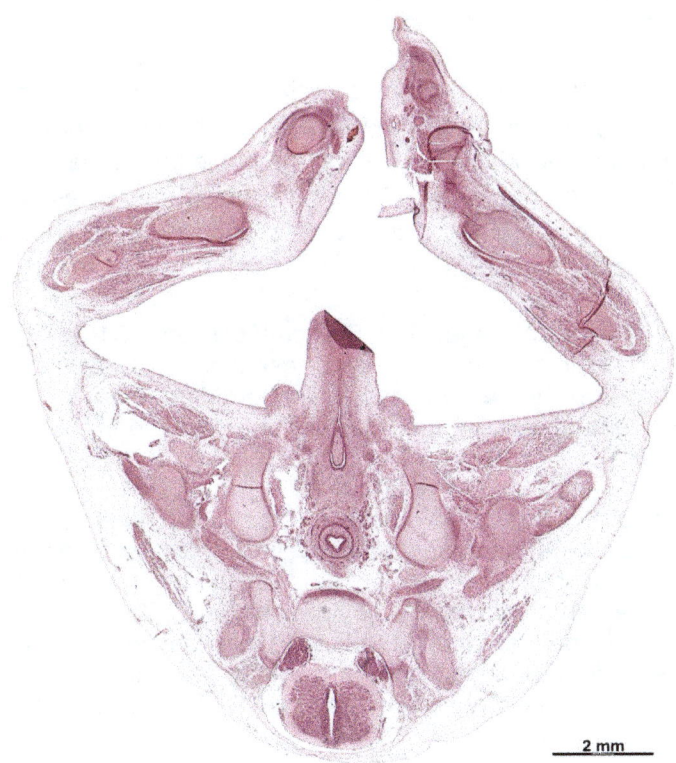

Speculation about the derivation of the genital tubercle

According to the new hypothesis, during the indifferent stages, the 5 sacral somites have to recede from their segmentation and disintegrate. The sclerotomes fuse to pelvic bones, which form the arcus, and they join together end-to-end in the midline of the ventral body with the pubic symphysis.

The 5 fused sacral myotomes with their genuine neurotomes (innervation) and angiotomes (vascularization), which are covered by dermatome growing below along the pubic bones, fuse together endways on the pubic area. These conjoined myotomes form the corpora cavernosa of the genital tubercle and follow the autonomic neuro-vascular bundles (Fig. V-5).

On the indifferent stages the 5 sacral somites (S1-S5) have to recede of their segmentation and desintegrate. The sclerotomes (grey color) fuse to pelvic bones, which form the arcus, they conjoin together end-to-end in the midline of ventral body with pubic symphysis.

The fused 5 sacral myotomes (M, red color) with its genuine neurotomes (blue) and angiotomes (yellow), covered by dermatome growing below along of pubic bones and fuse together endways on pubic area. The endwise conjoined myotomes form the corpora cavernosa of genital tubercle, following with dorsal neuro-vascular bundles (bold yellow and blue in the ring, labeled N). The top of myotomes ends become glans tubercle (G) covered of ectodermal layer.

During sexual differentiation: myotomes are forming the genital swelling (red), genital tubercle become glans penis or clitoridis, urogenital fold (green) originating from cloaca (hindgut) of embryo.

Female pattern or indifferent stage – small tubercle with opened vestibulum vaginae. The genital swellings form the labial folds; the branches of the genital tubercle (corpora cavernosa) surround the urogenital groove and located deep inside in the genital swellings.

Male pattern – fusion of labial folds into the urogenital sinus (or penile urethra) extends along the elongated phallus. The branches of the genital tubercle (corpora cavernosa) conjoin together.

Figure V-7. New theory about derivation of external genitalia (schematic).

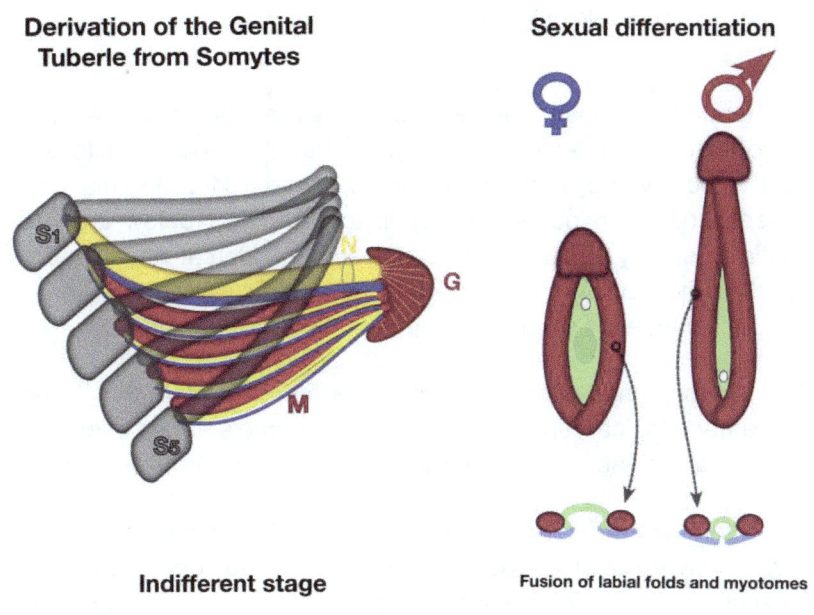

Derivation of the Genital Tuberle from Somytes

Sexual differentiation

Indifferent stage

Fusion of labial folds and myotomes

On the indifferent stages the 5 sacral somites (S1-S5) have to recede of their segmentation and desintegrate. The sclerotomes (gray color) fuse to pelvic bones, which form the arcus, they conjoin together end-to-end in the midline of the ventral body with pubic symphysis. The fused 5 sacral myotomes (M, red color) with their genuine neurotomes (blue) and angiotomes (yellow), covered by dermatome growing below along of pubic bones and fuse together at their ends in the pubic area. The conjoined myotomes form the corpora cavernosa, followed by dorsal neuro-vascular bundles (bold yellow and blue, labeled N). The top of myotomes ends becomes the glans tubercle (G) covered of ectodermal layer.

During sexual differentiation: myotomes are forming the genital swelling (red), genital tubercle becomes the glans penis or clitoridis, urogenital fold (green) originating from the cloaca (hindgut) of the embryo.

Female pattern or indifferent stage – small tubercle with opened vestibulum vaginae.

Male pattern – fusion of labial folds into the urogenital sinus (or penile urethra) extending along the elongated phallus.

The tops of the myotomes' ends become the glans tubercle, which is covered by an ectodermal layer. The glans penis (clitoris) is innervated by the somatic pudendal nerve (S1-S5). This nerve passes under the pubis symphysis to travel just below the Buck fascia to supply sensory innervation through dorsal neurovascular bundle. The neuronal axons terminate superficially on the glans of the genital tubercle's surface.

The sensory innervation maintains a segmental pattern that reflects the embryological origin of each dermatome's innervation. The genital neural tract originates from the sacral vertebral segments.

In the female embryo, the fused myotomes (analogues of the male corpora cavernosa) surround the vestibulum vaginae, forming the musculus bulbocavernosus and the ischiocavernosus deep in the genital swellings. Medially, they join into the glans clitoridis (same as the glans penis). The glans clitoridis has less surface area (compared to the glans penis), and thus the neurons are much tougher.

In the male embryo, the genital tubercle elongates and fuses to form the penis (phallus), and the genital swellings fuse to become the scrotum. The urogenital groove is transformed into the penile urethra, which terminates with an orificium on the glans penis.

The sclerotomes of 8-10 coccygeal pairs are reduced, and the myotomes form the pelvic diaphragm and striated muscles of the anus.

The genital tubercle derives from all of the following three germ layers:

- The glans of the tubercle (glans penis, clitoridis) is covered by ectoderm, which is derive from the apical ectodermal ridge.
- The corpora cavernosa derives from mesodermal somites.
- The urogenital groove originates from the cloacal endoderm (part of the hindgut), which forms the urethral plate epithelium.

During the undifferentiated stages, the early genital tubercle has a superficial affinity to the limb bud, but there is an important distinction between the two.

The upper limb buds derive from C3-Th1, while the lower limb buds derive from L2-S1 somitomeres. Whereas the limb bud is composed of mesoderm covered by surface ectoderm, the genital tubercle is derived from all three germ layers.

The genital tubercle derives from S1-S5 somitomeres and receives sensory innervation from the pudendal nerve, which provides the nervus dorsalis of the tubercle (penis and clitoridis).

The new theory is that the genital tubercle originates from conjoined genitogenous ribs, and this is the key difference between this process and limb budding.

It is likely that the initiation of derivation of the genital tubercle during the indifferent stages depends on growth factors that play a role in limb development from (5) sacral somitomeres. Signals for the development of genital somites derive from the notochord and neuromeres, which are stimulated by nerve growth factor. The apical ectodermal ridge (like in limb growth) exerts an inductive proliferation of the adjacent tubercle's mesoderm (corpora cavernosa). Androgens stimulate the masculinization of the indifferent genital tubercle by hypertrophy of the corpora cavernosa and through an inductive influence on the neurotomes with activation of nerve growth factor.

Patrick Tschopp et al. (2014) [29], Anna Herrera and Martin Cohn (2014) [30] considers, the paired genital swellings on either side of the cloacal membrane merge beneath the surface of ectoderm to form a single genital tubercle anterior to the cloaca.

I suppose, the genital swellings form the labial folds on females; they brought at the ventral midline and fuse together into the penile urethra on male embryo. The branches of the genital tubercle that derived from 5 fused myotomes (corpora cavernosa) surround the urogenital groove and located deep inside in the genital swellings.

The fusion of the labial folds into the urogenital sinus (or the penile urethra in the male embryo) extends along the elongated phallus. Typically, the process of elongation (outgrowth) of the genital tubercle and fusion of the urethral fold are proceeding together (like Prader stages). These processes may be discordant, as the genital tubercle (ectodermal and mesodermal) and the urogenital groove (endodermal) originate from different germ layers, and thus they are stimulated by different pathways of growth factors and receptors.

Erogenous sensitivity is perceived through numerous sensor neurons within the 5 sacral somitomeres. The embryonal precursors of genital erogenous sensation have principal differences: the glans clitoridis (penis) has somatic sensitivity through the nervus dorsalis clitoridis (penis) from 5 sacral S1-S5 neurotomes; while the corpora cavernosa has autonomic innervation from pudendal nerves, that provide the erectile function; and the vestibulum (female) vaginae and (male) penile urethra have visceral innervation originating from the hindgut. The hymen is a mucous membrane located between the fused mesonephric ducts and the urogenital sinus (part of the cloaca), and it has high sensitivity originating from the autonomic and visceral nervous systems. The clitoris, vestibulum vaginae, and hymenal fold are erotically important organs that contribute to female erogenous sensation, arousal and orgasm. 28

Presumably, sexual differentiation of external genitalia is final in gender embryogenesis, but surprisingly derivation of the indifferent genital tubercle from 5 sacral somites occurs before gonadal and internal organs development.

References

1. Sadler TW. "Langman`s Medical Embryology". XII-th edn, Baltimore: Lippincott Williams&Wilkins, 2012; 232-259.

2. Hill MA. Embryology BGD Lecture - Sexual Differentiation. Retrieved October 16, 2014. URL: http://php.med.unsw.edu.au/embryology/index.php?title=BGD_Lecture_-_Sexual_Differentiation

3. Jost AA. The new look at the mechanism controlling sex differentiation in mammals. John Hopkins Medical Journal 1972; 130: 28-36.

4. Wilhelm D, Palmer S, Koopman P. Sex determination and gonadal development in mammals. Physiol. Rev.: 2007, 87(1);1-28 PubMed 17237341| Physiol. Rev. doi: 10.1152/physrev.00009.2006

5. Cohn MJ. Development of the external genitalia: conserved and divergent mechanisms of appendage patterning. Dev. Dyn.: 2011, 240(5);1108-15 PubMed 21465625. doi: 10.1002/dvdy.22631.

6. Munger SC, Natarajan A, Looger LL, Ohler U, Capel B. Fine time course expression analysis identifies cascades of activation and repression and maps a putative regulator of mammalian sex determination. PLoS Genet.: 2013, 9(7);e1003630 PubMed 23874228. doi: 10.1371/journal.pgen.1003630.

7. Mieszczak J, Houk CP, Lee PA. Assignment of the sex of rearing in the neonate with a disorder of sex development. Curr Opin Pediatr. 2009;21:541-547. doi: 10.1097/MOP.0b013e32832c6d2c.

8. Sax L. How common is intersex?: a response to Anne Fausto-Sterling. J Sex Res. 2002;39:174-178.

9. Hughes IA, Houk C, Ahmed SF, et al. Consensus statement on management of intersex disorders. Archives of Disease in Childhood, 2006; 91, 554–563. doi.org/10.1136/adc.2006.098319

10. Cools, M., Nordenström, A., Robeva, R. et al. Caring for individuals with a difference of sex development (DSD): a Consensus Statement. Nat Rev Endocrinol 14, 415–429 (2018). https://doi.org/10.1038/s41574-018-0010-8.

11. Pasterski V, Prentice P, Hughes IA et al. Consequences of the Chicago consensus on disorders of sex development (DSD): current practices in Europe. Archives of Disease in Childhood, 2010; 95, 618–623. doi:10.1136/adc.2009.163840
12. Houk CP, Lee PA. Update on disorders of sex development. Curr Opin Endocrinol Diabetes Obes, 2012; 19:28-32. doi: 10.1097/MED.0b013e32834edacb
13. Ahmed F, Achermann J, Arlt W, et al. UK guidance on the initial evaluation of an infant or an adolescent with a suspected disorder of sex development. Clin Endocrinol (Oxf). 2011 July; 75(1): 12–26. doi: 10.1111/j.1365-2265.2011.04076.x
14. Ahmed SF, Gardner M, Sandberg DE. Management of children with disorders of sex development: new care standards explained. Psychology and Sexuality, January 2014; 5(1): 5-14. doi: 10.1080/19419899.2013.831211
15. Prader A. Der genitalbefund beim pseudohermaproditus feminus des kongenitalen adrenogenitalen syndromes. Helv Pediatr Acta.: 1954, 9; 231-248.
16. Prader A, Gurtner HP. The syndrome of male pseudohermaphrodism in congenital adrenocortical hyperplasia without overproduction of androgens (adrenal male pseudohermaphrodism). Helv. Paediatr. Acta.: 1955, 10; 397-412.
17. Creighton SM. Long-term outcome of feminization surgery: the London experience. BJU 2004; Int 200493(suppl. 3)44–46.46. doi:10.1111/j.1464-410X.2004.04708.x
18. Sugiyama Y, Mizuno H, Hayashi Y, Imamine H, Ito T, Kato I, Yamamoto-Tomita M, Aoyama M, Asai K, Togari H. Severity of virilization of external genitalia in Japanese patients with salt-wasting 21-hydroxylase deficiency. Tohoku J Exp Med. 2008 Aug;215(4):341-8. doi.org/10.1620/tjem.215.341
19. Makiyan Z. Studies of gonadal sex differentiation. Organogenesis 2016; 12(1):42-51. doi:10.1080/15476278.2016.1145318
20. Makiyan Z New theory of uterovaginal embryogenesis. Organogenesis. 2016 2016; 12(1):33-41. doi:10.1080/15476278.2016.1145317

21. Oppelt P, Renner SP, Brucker S, et al. The VCUAM (Vagina Cervix Uterus Adnex-associated Malformation) classification: a new classification for genital malformations. Fertil Steril. 2005 Nov;84(5):1493-7. doi:10.1016/j.fertnstert.2005.05.036

22. Grimbizis GF1, Gordts S, Di Spiezio Sardo A, et al. The ESHRE/ESGE consensus on the classification of female genital tract congenital anomalies. Hum Reprod. 2013 Aug;28(8):2032-44. doi: 10.1093/humrep/det098.

23. Wittekind C, Greene FL, Hutter RVP, et al. TNM atlas: illustrated guide to the TNM/pTNM classification of malignant tumours (5th ed.), Springer, Heidelberg. 2004

24. Lin C, Yin Y, Veith GM, et al. Temporal and spatial dissection of Shh signaling in genital tubercle development. Development. 2009; 136(23);3959-67 PubMed 19906863. doi: 10.1242/dev.039768.

25. Petiot A, Perriton CL, Dickson C, Cohn MJ. Development of the mammalian urethra is controlled by Fgfr2-IIIb. Development 2005; 132:2441–2450.

26. Yang JH, Menshenina J, Cunha GR, et al. Morphology of mouse external genitalia: implications for a role of estrogen in sexual dimorphism of the mouse genital tubercle. J Urol. 2010; 184:1604–1609.

27. Sinnecker GH, Hiort O, Dibbelt L, et al. Phenotypic classification of male pseudohermaphroditism due to steroid 5 alphareductase 2 deficiency. Am J Med Genet. 1996; 63:223–230.

28. Makiyan Z. Female sexuality. Lulu Publisning, USA. 2013 ISBN-9781304000125. http://www.lulu.com/shop/zohrab-makiyan/female-sexuality/ebook/product-21025371.html

29. Tschopp P, Sherratt E, Sanger TJ, et al. A relative shift in cloacal location repositions external genitalia in amniote evolution. Nature. 2014 Dec 18;516(7531):391-4. doi: 10.1038/nature13819.

30. Herrera AM, Cohn MJ. Embryonic origin and compartmental organization of the external genitalia. Scientific Reports 2014; 4:6896 doi: 10.1038/srep06896

VI. SYSTEMATIZATION FOR FEMALE GENITAL VARIATIONS

Early recognition and classification of uterovaginal malformations is important to ensure appropriate management before clinical symptoms and complications develop.

The European Society of Human Reproduction and Embryology (ESHRE) and the European Society for Gynaecological Endoscopy (ESGE) have published a consensus statement on the classification of female genital tract variations that focuses on uterovaginal malformations only, and distinguishes 6 classes of uterine variations in combination with cervical and vaginal defects (Grimbizis et al., 2016). This classification does not identify all possible variations and does not consider all elements of urogenital development.

Hence, the unified Systematization for Female Genital Anatomic Variations (Table VI-1) was developed, considering all female genital organ malformations, and corresponding to chronologic embryological stages. These new classifications provide complete diagnostic patterns of female genital variations by investigation of the genome (karyotype), gonadal morphology, internal genital anatomy, and external genital virilization stages.

The female reproductive tract is composed of gonads (primary) that contain gametes; an internal reproductive tract (including the fallopian tubes, uterus and vagina); and external genitalia. Disorders of sex development (DSD) may affect any of these organs. The gonadal morphology and appropriate surgery for patients with DSD are described in "Studies of gonadal sex differentiation" (Makiyan, 2016a).

Congenital malformations of the vulva, including fusion of the labial or clitoral hypertrophy, are seen in DSD and severe virilization of the external genitalia, as discussed in the "Systematization of ambiguous genitalia" Makiyan, 2016b).

Table VI-1. An example of a unified Systematization for Female Genital Variations (Anomalies).

Nosology	Karyotype (genome)	Gonadal morphology	Internal Anatomy	External genital virilization stages	Surgical treatment
Uterovaginal aplasia	46,XX	ovary	non-functional rudiments (type 1-a)	female	Creation of neovagina.
Uterovaginal aplasia	46,XX	ovary	uterine rudiments, functional (type 1-b)	female	Laparoscopy, removal of the uterine rudiments. Creation of neovagina.
Turner syndrome, classic form	45,X	fibrous streak gonad	uterine rudiments, non-functional (1-a)	female	Laparoscopy, removal of the uterine rudiments. Creation of neovagina.
Turner syndrome, mosaicism	45,X/46,XX	ovarian dysgenesis	uterine rudiments, functional (type 1-b)	female	Laparoscopy, removal of the uterine rudiments. Creation of neovagina.
Turner syndrome, mosaicism	45,X/46,XY	fibrous streak, testicular dysgenesis, ovotestis	uterine rudiments, non-functional (1-a)	ambiguous genitalia (virilization degree I-IV by Prader)	laparoscopy gonadectomy; feminizing plasty. Creation of neovagina.
46,XY gonadal dysgenesis, incomplete form	46,XY	testicular dysgenesis	uterine rudiments (1-a, 1-b), hypoplastic uterus (type11) and vagina	ambiguous genitalia (virilization degree I-V by Prader)	Laparoscopy gonadectomy; feminizing plasty.

46,XY gonadal dysgenesis, complete form	46,XY	testicular dysgenesis	hypoplastic (type 11) or normal uterus and vagina	female	Laparoscopy gonadectomy.
Androgen insensitivity syndrome, incomplete form	46,XY	testicles	uterine rudiments, non-functional (1-a)	ambiguous genitalia (virilization degree I-V by Prader)	Laparoscopy gonadectomy; feminizing plasty: clitororeduction, introitoplasty.
Androgen insensitivity syndrome, complete form	46,XY	testicles	uterine rudiments, non-functional (1-a)	female	Laparoscopy gonadectomy; Feminizing plasty, Creation of neovagina.
Ovotesticular DSD	46,XY; 46,XX/46,XY	ovotestis	uterine rudiments, non-functional (1-a)	ambiguous genitalia (virilization degree I-IV by Prader)	Laparoscopy gonadectomy; feminizing plasty: clitororeduction, introitoplasty. Creation of neovagina.
Congenital adrenal hyperplasia	46.XX	ovary	normal uterus or uterovaginal anomalies (type 4-11)	ambiguous genitalia (virilization degree I-V by Prader)	Feminizing plasty. Laparoscopic surgery, according to uterovaginal anomalies.
Uterovaginal anomalies	46,XX	ovary	Type 1-11 (in tab. 1)	female	According to anomalous type

VII. NEW INSIGHTS INTO THE EMBRYOGENESIS OF THE FEMALE REPRODUCTIVE SYSTEM

Considering, the congenital anatomic (structural) variations of the reproductive system are defined as deviations from normal embryogenesis; each anatomic variant corresponds to persistent developmental stages.

A systematic comparison between reproductive organ maldevelopment and contemporary embryological investigations, together with an in-depth literature review, has revealed the existence of many disagreements and controversies surrounding the embryogenesis of the female reproductive system.

This new insight offers a cardinally different representation of the reproductive organ morphogenesis from that of the current view, at all its consequent stages.

Consequently, the idea of formulating a new theory of embryonic morphogenesis, including gonadal sex differentiation, uterovaginal morphogenesis, and derivation of the genital tubercle, was stimulated (Makiyan 2016; Makiyan 2017). This new theory offers a cardinally different representation of the reproductive organ's morphogenesis from that of the current view, at all its consequent stages.

Fig. VII-1. New insights into the embryogenesis of the female reproductive system. Schematic pattern.

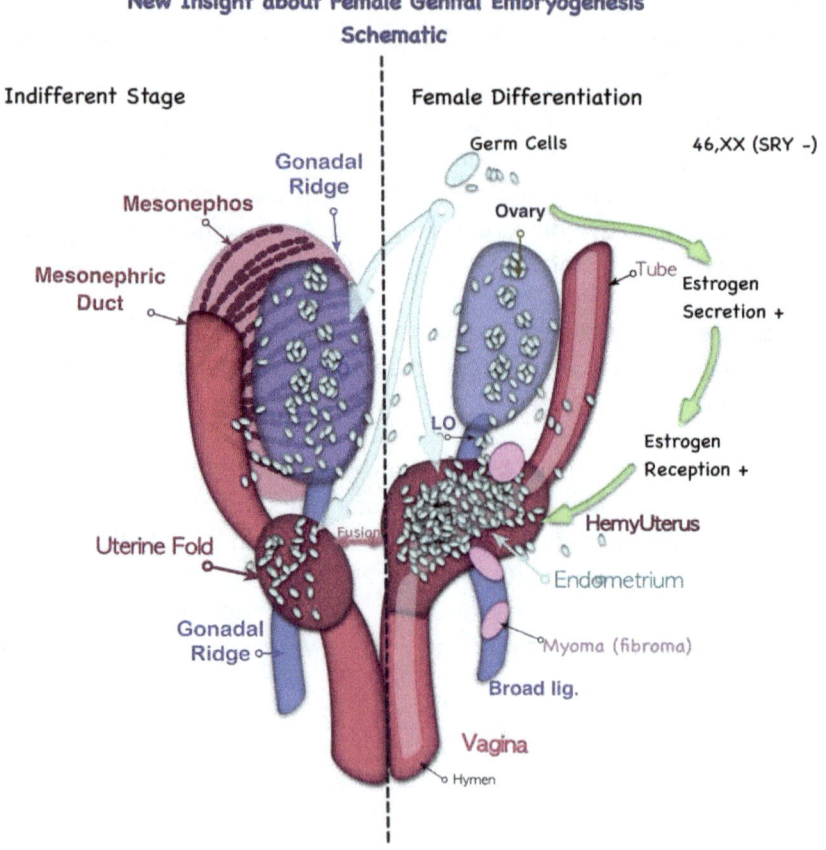

New theory of female sex organ's development

(Fig. VII-1)

1. The genome is a determinative factor for sex differentiation, despite X and Y chromosomes are being homologous. Sex determinative factors are numerous, some of them are also located in somatic chromosomes.

2. Primordial germ cells migrate from the hypoblast to the gonadal ridges, which later derive into the germline epithelium of the ovary, the ovarian ligament, the uterine broad ligament, and the eutopic endometrium. Ectopic primordial germ cells might transform into heterotopic endometria within the migration pathway.

3. Gonadal sex differentiation depends on the derivation of the embryonic urinary system (mesonephros) and it is not solely governed by *SRY*. Nevertheless, the *SRY* gene has a primary role in sex differentiation, through exerting an inductive influence on the mesonephros, e.g., inducing cell migration and proliferation, and organogenesis.

   Cell proliferation in the mesonephric system, to form tubules and corpuscles, stimulates the masculinization of the gonad into testes. On the contrary, a reduction of the mesonephric tubular system results in female gonad development into ovaries.

   An intermediate developmental stage during gonadal embryogenesis, in which both the male and the female gonads were represented by both testicular and ovarian tissues, would result in the formation of an ovotestis. This intermediate organ could be the key for a full understanding of the ambiguous gonad´s developmental origin (which is presently unknown).

Nevertheless, the provisory urinary system of the embryo, formed by the pronephros and the mesonephros, has a primary derivative role in gonadal sex differentiation.

4. Hormonal stage. In the male pathway, testes (Leydig cells) secrete androgens that mediate the virilization of both the internal and external organs whereas. In the female pathway, ovaries secrete oestrogens that stimulate the feminizing development of indifferent organs, both internal and external. Androgen and oestrogen receptors' sensitivity plays a fundamental role in these processes.

An androgen deficiency causes abnormalities in male organ development, such as those seen in 46,XY disorders of sex development: testicular dysgenesis syndrome and defects in androgen receptor's sensitivity leading to androgen-insensitivity syndrome.

Oestrogen deficiencies and oestrogen insensitivity are manifested as congenital uterovaginal anomalies, which persist along different embryonic developmental stages, such as uterovaginal aplasia, doubling uterus, and septate uterus.

The mesonephric ducts (which first appear as ureters of the mesonephros) form the fallopian tubes and the vagina. Additionally, the uterus is formed in the area in which the mesonephric ducts intersect with the gonadal ridges. Hence, the female reproductive tract originates from the provisionary or temporal urinary tract.

Noteworthy, the paramesonephric ducts do not exist. Here, an important question should be asked: What is the anti-Müllerian hormone (AMH) for?

There are two main processes leading to the uterine organogenesis. First, tissues in the intersection between the gonadal ridges and the mesonephral ducts are forming the uterine folds with an endometrial cavity, where polypotent germ cells have differentiate and grow into the myometrial and endometrial layers. Second, both uterine folds fuse together to form the normal uterus (having just one cavity). These processes may explain the morphological differences between uterine myometrial layers and the wall of the fallopian tubes, as well as the presence of eutopic endometrium inside of the uterine folds.

Possible aetiologies of congenital uterine malformations may be: X-monosomy, failure in the oestrogen influence over undifferentiated organs, insensitivity of the oestrogen receptors of indifferent organs, oestrogen-dependent developmental insufficiency, and insulin-like growth factors.

5. External genitalia originate from the genital tubercle and genital swellings. The indifferent genital tubercle develops early, in the 3rd week of gestation, from 5 sacral somites, earlier than gonadal and internal organ development. These sacral somites must recede from their segmentation and disintegrate: the sclerotomes form the pelvic bones, the fused myotomes following with their genuine neurotomes and the angiotomes attach to to the corpora cavernosa (Fig. VII-2).

In the female embryo, the fused myotomes (analogues of the male corpora cavernosa) surrounding the vestibulum vaginae form the musculus bulbocavernosus and the musculus ischiocavernosus, deep inside ofm the genital swellings. Medially, these muscles move into the glans clitoridis (in the same way as they move into the glans penis). The glans clitoridis has less surface area than the glans penis; therefore its neuron terminal concentration is much higher.

In the male embryo, the genital tubercle elongates and fuses to form the penis (phallus), and the genital swellings fuse to become the scrotum. The urogenital groove is transformed into the penile urethra, which terminates with an orificium on the glans penis.

Typically, the process of elongation (outgrowth) of the genital tubercle and the fusion of the urethral fold proceed simultaneously. These processes may be discordant because the genital tubercle (ectodermal and mesodermal) and the urogenital groove (endodermal) originate from different germ layers. Thus, they are stimulated by different pathways.

Ambiguity (intersexuality) of external genital anatomy in 46,XY patients results from failures in androgen hormone influence over undifferentiated organs and from altered receptor sensitivity; in 46,XX females, it is the result of an androgen excess.

Clinical and experimental evidences

1. Clinical cases of sex reversal of 46,XX (SRY-negative) male syndrome, especially those with normal spermatozoa and testes, are controversial to the classic concept of sex differentiation. The genotype of somatic cells (epithelial or leucocytes) and of the gonadal germline epithelium is sometimes different, due to mosaicism or chimerism (Makiyan 2016).

2. Primordial germ cells at an early stage (during migration) do not have sex specific characteristics. Still, primordial germ cells that reach gonadal ridges, which develop into the gonads, the ligamentum ovarii, and the broad ligament, may persist in situ and grow into benign (leiomyoma, fibroma, and endometriosis) or malignant tumors, even in fetuses (Signorile and Baldi 2020).

3. According to histological images of human female embryos on Carnegie stage 13 (approximately at the 4th week of development), mesonephral ducts are located at the paramedial sides, and paramesonephral ducts do not exist (Hill 2019b).

   Moreover, images from Carnegie stage 22 (approximately at the 8th week of development) also show the mesonephral ducts at the paramedial sides. Here, the medial paramesonephral ducts potentially correspond to genital ridges (Hill 2019c).

4. In the 9th edition of Langman's Medical Embryology (Sadler 2004; p. 324, Fig. 14.3-C), there is an electron micrograph of a female embryo in the same (early) stage of development, where it is possible to see the genital ridges growing immediately below the gonads and that the mesonephral ducts are located at the paramedial sides of the mesonephros and they conjoin together. It is also possible to observe that at the intersection zone between the mesonephral ducts and the gonadal ridges the uterine folds are being formed. The picture of an early stage of embryonic development corresponds to the anatomy of an uterovaginal aplasia, where the uterine rudiments detected at the area of intersection between fallopian tubes with broad and ovarian ligaments (fig. 1). A unique clinical of congenital uterovaginal aplasia revealed in young female patient (fig. 1.) Laparoscopically, multiple myoma have been detected in the both nonfunctional uterine rudiments.

   Dr. Christopher Hurst et al. (2002) investigated in utero the effects of the exposure to a teratogenic compound during the critical periods of female rat's organogenesis and found that there was a disruption in early morphogenesis by increasing the distance between the unfused Müllerian ducts. They also found evidences of uterine fold development in the intersection area between the mesonephral ducts and the gonadal ridges and of the fusion of both uterine folds together.

Furthermore, Dr. Hashimoto (2003), observing samples from gonadal early stages of development by electron microscopy, detected an active cell-to-cell communication between Müllerian and Wolffian cells.

The Müllerian theory (1830) represented a great progress in the biological sciences when it was proposed, back in 1830. It was also a remarkable accomplishment since Müller investigated the human embryo by using simple light microscopy. However, studies done by electronic microscopy revealed that the paramedial ducts (the so called Müllerian ducts) are, in reality, the mesonephric ducts. According to the new theory, the medial or Wolffian ducts correspond to the gonadal ridges, whereas the paramedial or Müllerian ducts coincide with the mesonephral ducts. Finally, it proposes that paramesonephral ducts do not exist.

5. The tips of the myotomes, at one of their ends, fuse and become the glans tubercle, which is covered by an ectodermal layer (fig. 2). Both the glans penis and the glans clitoridis are innervated by the somatic pudendal nerve. The 5 fused sacral myotomes preserve their genuine neurotomes (innervation) and angiotomes (vascularization). The sensory innervation maintains a segmental pattern that reflects the embryological origin of each dermatome's innervation. The genital neural tract originates from the S1-S5 sacral vertebral segments. The nerve passes under the pubic symphysis to supply sensory innervation through the dorsal neurovascular bundle. The neuronal axons terminate superficially in the glans of the genital tubercle's surface (Makiyan 2017).

Conclusion

The new theory proposes that gonadal sex differentiation depends on the inductive influence of the mesonephros, together with SRY. The proliferation of the mesonephric system, tubules and corpuscles, stimulates the masculinization of the gonads into testes. Whereas, its reduction results in female gonadal development. The mesonephric ducts form the fallopian tubes and the vagina.

The uterus develops in the crossing area between the mesonephric ducts and the gonadal ridges, where the polypotent germ cells differentiate and grow, forming the myometrial and endometrial layers. The genital tubercle originates from 5 conjoined sacral somites, likely as limb budding, preserving their genuine innervation and vascularization.

This new systematic evaluation will be necessary for future embryologic investigations. The proposed theory may be the key for understanding the etiopathogenesis of genital anomalies; major gynaecological diseases, comma leiomyoma and endometriosis from polypotential germ cells.

This new insight, leading to the proposal of a new theory, may be able to explain the normal pathway followed during female genital embryogenesis as well as the maldevelopment stages which result in congenital anomalies.

The proposed origin of both eutopic endometrial and myometrial layers from polypotent primordial germ cells in the female embryo, disseminated at indifferent stages, and their persistence within the uterine folds, may be the key for understanding the aetiology of female genital anomalies and major benign gynaecological diseases, comma leiomyoma and endometriosis, explaining their morphology, pathogenesis and localization.

Fig. VII-2. Laparoscopy in a young patient with complete uterine and vaginal aplasia. The nonfunctional uterine rudiments, without an endometrial cavity, detected in the crossing area between Fallopian tubes with ovarian and broad ligaments.

Multiple myoma revealed in the both uterine rudiments, despite there are nonfunctional.

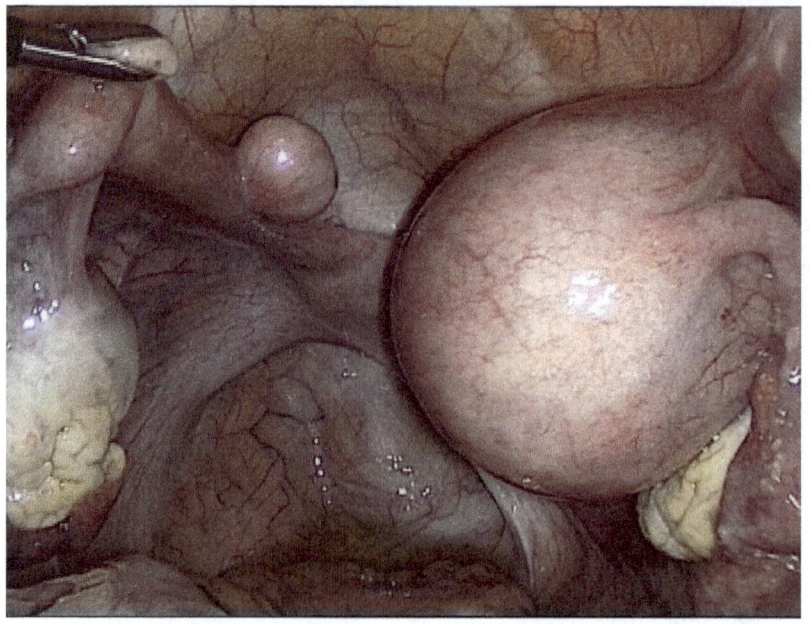

References

Batista RL. (2019) Complete Androgen Insensitivity in Girls with Inguinal Hernias: A Serendipity Opportunity for Early Diagnosis. J Invest Surg. Aug 9:1-2. doi: 10.1080/08941939.2019.1612970. Epub ahead of print.

Cunha GR, Kurita T, Cao M, Shen J, Robboy S & Baskin L. (2017). Molecular mechanisms of development of the human fetal female reproductive tract. Differentiation. 97, 54-72. doi.org/10.1016/j.diff.2017.07.003

Signorile P.G., Baldi A. (2020) The Presence of Endometriosis in the Human Fetus. In: Nezhat C.H. (eds) Endometriosis in Adolescents. Springer, Cham. https://doi.org/10.1007/978-3-030-52984-0_8

Fritsch, H., Hoermann, R., Bitsche, M., Pechriggl, E. & Reich, O. (2013) Development of epithelial and mesenchymal regionalization of the human fetal utero-vaginal anlagen. J Anat, 222, 462 – 472.

Hashimoto R. (2003) Development of the human Müllerian duct in the sexually undifferentiated stage. Anat Rec A Discov Mol Cell Evol Biol. 272(2):514-9.

Herrera AM, Cohn MJ. (2014) Embryonic origin and compartmental organization of the external genitalia. Scientific Reports. 4:68-96. http://dx.doi.org/10.1038/srep06896

Hill MA. (2019a) Embryology Primordial Germ Cell Migration Movie. Retrieved from https://embryology.med.unsw.edu.au/embryology/index.php/Primordial_Germ_Cell_Migration_Movie#Mouse_E9.0_Primordial_Germ_Cell_Migration

Hill MA. (2019b) Embryology Stage 13 image 093.jpg. Retrieved from https://embryology.med.unsw.edu.au/embryology/index.php/File:Stage_13_image_093.jpg

Hill MA. (2019c) Embryology Stage 22 image 214.jpg. https://embryology.med.unsw.edu.au/embryology/index.php/File:Stage_22_image_214.jpg

Hurst CH, Abbott B, Schmid JE, Birnbaum LS. (2002) Feulgen staining of female rat reproductive tracts after GD 15 administration of 1.0 µg TCDD/kg showing width of interductal mesenchyme. Toxicol Sci

Published online:; 65(1). Available from URL: https://academic.oup.com/view-large/figure/24474822/120120928006.gif

Jost A. (1972) A new look at the mechanism controlling sex differentiation in mammals. Johns Hopkins Med J. 130,28-36

Makiyan Z. (2016) Studies of gonadal sex differentiation. Organogenesis. 12(1):42-51. doi.org/10.1080/15476278.2016.1145318

Makiyan Z. (2017) Systematization of ambiguous genitalia. Organogenesis. 12(4):169-82; doi.org/10.1080/15476278.2016.1210749

Makiyan Z. (2020) Systematization for female genital anatomic variations [published online ahead of print, 2020 Aug 11]. Clin Anat. 2020;10.1002/ca.23668. doi:10.1002/ca.23668

Müller JP (1830). Bildungsgeschichte der Genitalien Düsseldorf: Arnz, pp 185-187

Nistal M, García-Fernández E, Mariño-Enríquez A, et al. (2007) Usefulness of gonadal biopsy in the diagnosis of sexual developmental disorders. Actas Urol Esp. 31(9):1056-75. http://dx.doi.org/10.1016/S0210-4806(07)73767-1

Robboy, S.J., Kurita, T., Baskin, L. & Cunha, G.R. (2017) New insights into human female reproductive tract development. Differentiation, 97, 9 – 22.

Sadler TW. "Langman's Medical Embryology." (2004) IX-th edn Baltimore: Lippincott Williams&Wilkins; p. 324, Fig. 14.3-C.

Tschopp P, Sherratt E, Sanger T, Groner A, Aspiras A, Hu J, Pourqui1e O, Gros J, Tabin C. (2014) A relative shift in cloacal location repositions external genitalia in amniote evolution. Nature. 516(7531):391-4. http://dx.doi.org/10.1038/nature-13819

Wilhelm D, Palmer S & Koopman P. (2007). Sex determination and gonadal development in mammals. Physiol. Rev. 87, 1-28. doi.org/10.1152/physrev.00009.2006

Abbreviations

AIS - adrenal insensitivity syndrome

AMH – anti-Mullerian hormone

DSD – disorders of sex development

EUROCAT - European Surveillance of Congenital Anomalies

MIS - Mullerian inhibitory substance

MRI – magnetic resonance imaging

PMDS - Persistent Mullerian duct syndrome

SRY – sex-determining region Y

Front cover art image

The red image on the front cover is a symbol of female (f), sex (sx), extraordinary (x) and dual origin of gender with masculine derivation.

Author page

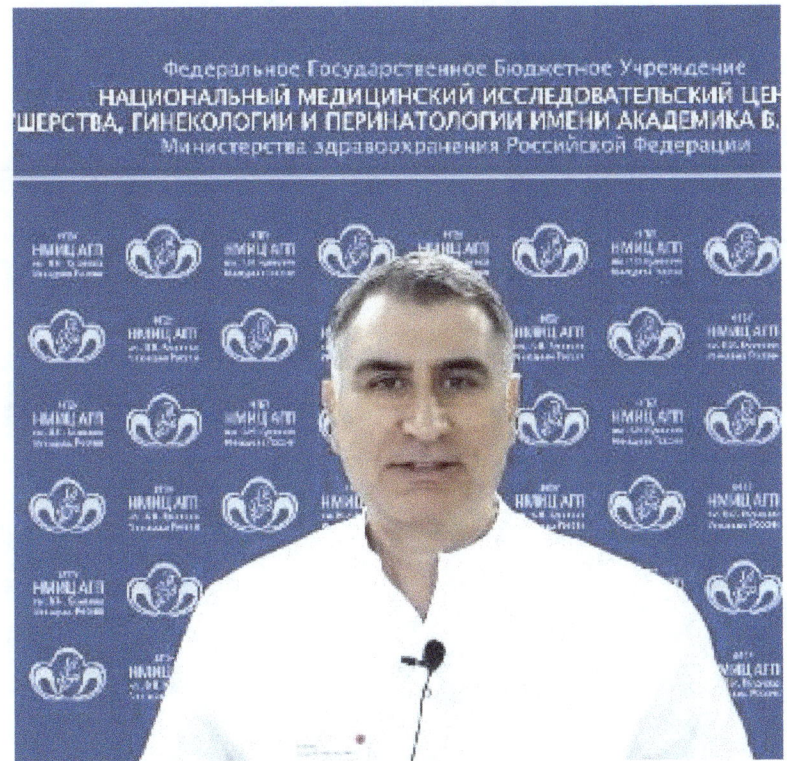

Zohrab Makiyan, doctor of medicine, practicing surgeon-gynecologist, focused on surgical correction of female genital anomalies, endometriosis and plastic surgery.
Principal scientist, working at the department of operative gynecology at Federal State National Medical Research Center of Obstetrics, Gynecology and Perinatology in Moscow, Russia.

Email: zorroh@icloud.com, makiyan@mail.ru

www.ingramcontent.com/pod-product-compliance
Lightning Source LLC
Chambersburg PA
CBHW060856170526
45158CB00001B/379